IMAGES
of America

GRIFFIN MEMORIAL HOSPITAL

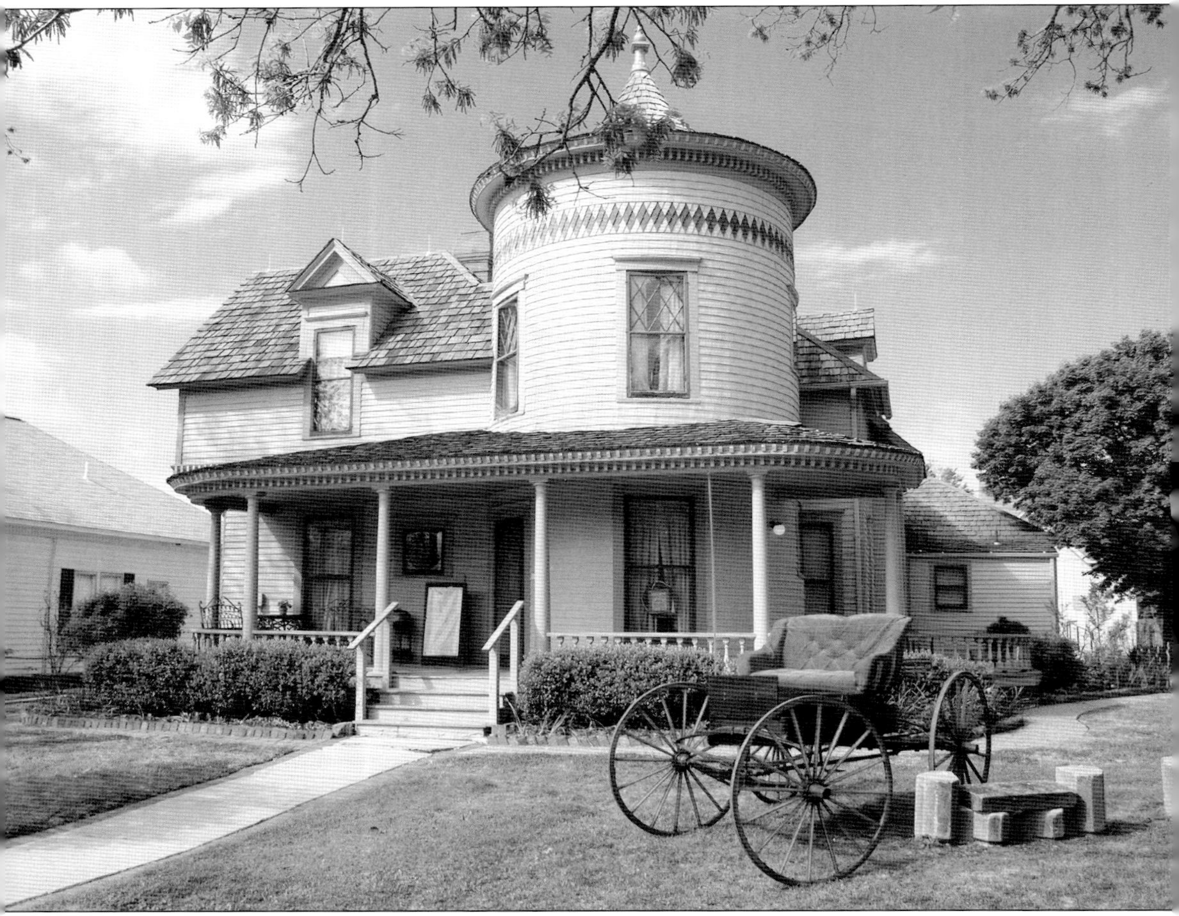

The Moore-Lindsay Historical House Museum is located in Norman, Oklahoma, and is operated by the Cleveland County Historical Society. (Cleveland County Historical Society.)

On the Cover: Griffin Memorial Hospital's first structure was the administration and classroom building for High Gate College, a college for women that was established by the Southern Methodist Church in 1890, one year after the settlement of Norman. The college only lasted for five years. In 1895, the Oklahoma Sanitarium Company bought High Gate College, and in 1915, the State of Oklahoma bought the Oklahoma Sanitarium Company and established Central State Hospital. (Oklahoma Historical Society.)

IMAGES
of America

GRIFFIN MEMORIAL HOSPITAL

Suzanne H. Schrems, PhD,
on behalf of the
Cleveland County Historical Society

ARCADIA
PUBLISHING

ISBN 978-1-4671-0697-9

Published by Arcadia Publishing
Charleston, South Carolina

Printed in the United States of America

Library of Congress Control Number: 2021935295

For all general information, please contact Arcadia Publishing:
Telephone 843-853-2070
Fax 843-853-0044
E-mail sales@arcadiapublishing.com
For customer service and orders:
Toll-Free 1-888-313-2665

Visit us on the Internet at www.arcadiapublishing.com

This book is dedicated to those who found mental wellness through the treatments and programs initiated at Griffin Memorial in the early to mid-20th century.

Contents

Acknowledgments		6
Introduction		7
1.	From College to Asylum: 1890–1914	9
2.	Growth of an Institution: 1915–1939	29
3.	Misery and Overcrowding: 1940s	51
4.	A New Era: 1950s	71
5.	More Changes: 1950s	89
6.	The Era of Dr. Hayden Donahue: 1960s	107

Acknowledgments

There are very few buildings left on the grounds of Griffin Memorial Hospital. The Oklahoma Department of Health still operates part of the hospital, and there are still programs to treat people with varying degrees of mental illness. There are also programs at Griffin for those with drug or alcohol addictions. Because of the private nature of mental illness, it was not possible to tour the buildings that still exist, including the American Legion Memorial Chapel and Hope Hall. Most of the photographs in this book are from the archives at the Oklahoma Historical Society. Photograph archivist Rachel Mosman was very efficient and helpful in compiling the many images that were obtained in several different phases. Also, I want to thank Vicky Johnson Photography for capturing, in black-and-white photographs, the elements of the buildings that still grace the Griffin Memorial Hospital grounds today. Most of the historical information that accompanies the photographs comes from articles found at Newspapers.com, especially in regard to the photographs from the *Daily Oklahoman* collection. The board of the Cleveland County Historical Society has been very supportive of this book and the two previous books that I authored for Arcadia Publishing, *Norman: 1889–1949* and *Norman's Navy Years: 1942–1959.* All author proceeds from these books go to the Cleveland County Historical Society for the care of the Moore-Lindsay Historic House Museum.

The following abbreviations are used in courtesy lines throughout the book to indicate which organization provided the associated image: Cleveland County Historical Society (CCHS) and Oklahoma Historical Society (OHS).

INTRODUCTION

Many people who live in Norman or the surrounding area worked at Griffin Memorial Hospital as patient attendants, maintenance personnel, cooks, laundry attendants, or part of the professional staff of nurses and doctors. Others who grew up in Norman have watched the growth of Griffin Memorial over the years and also witnessed the decline of the institution. New residents who moved to Norman as the town expanded knew little about Griffin Memorial Hospital until a Walmart was established across the street. Customers became curious about the empty space, especially the American Legion Memorial Chapel that stands as a sentinel towering over what was once a busy institution.

Griffin Memorial Hospital was established in 1895, when the Oklahoma Sanitarium Company purchased High Gate College. The college was established by the Indian Mission Annual Conference of the Southern Methodist Church in cooperation with the leading citizens of Norman. It stood on a slight rise at the end of East Main Street on land donated by C.J. Bowling just outside the city limits. High Gate College was the first school of higher education in Oklahoma Territory. It survived for only five years. In 1892, the territorial legislature designated Norman for a territorial university, which became the University of Oklahoma. High Gate College found it difficult to compete with the tuition-free territorial university, and the women's college closed its doors in 1895. Shortly before Oklahoma Sanitarium Company purchased the High Gate College building, the company secured a contract from the Oklahoma territorial legislature. The company continued to receive legislative funding until 1915, when the State of Oklahoma bought the failing sanitarium; the new state institution was renamed Central State Hospital and was intended to serve the central Oklahoma region. Western State Hospital in Fort Supply and Eastern State Hospital in Vinita served the mentally ill in their respective locations.

Central State Hospital was under the supervision of Dr. David W. Griffin, who began his career in mental health with the Oklahoma Sanitarium Company in 1899. Griffin became superintendent of Central State Hospital in 1910. At that time, there were 325 patients in the hospital. Griffin successfully worked with the Oklahoma legislature to obtain funding for the hospital and for the expansion of new buildings. However, housing did not keep up with the numbers of patients entering the hospital each year. By the 1950s, there were close to 3,000 patients at Central State Hospital. Griffin held what was then a new philosophy about the treatment of the mentally ill. He believed that many of those who were institutionalized suffered from minor mental problems, and with proper treatment, they could leave the hospital. Griffin did not like the stigma associated with mental illness and believed that it should be recognized and treated in the same manner as doctors approached other illnesses. Even though Griffin worked well with Oklahoma legislators, for the 50 years that he was superintendent of the hospital, it lacked the funds needed for sufficient patient housing, attendants, and professional staff. In his tenure at Central State Hospital, Griffin accomplished what he could with the little funding the hospital received. His legacy includes the establishment of the veteran's hospital at the southeast corner of the property. Dr. Griffin retired in 1950. After his death in 1953, the Oklahoma legislature renamed the place where he worked for over half a century Central State Griffin Memorial Hospital, better known today as Griffin Memorial Hospital.

By 1960, under the supervision of Dr. Hayden Donahue, a new approach to mental illness was introduced at Griffin Memorial. Donahue worked as a physician in North Africa during World War II. Along with another doctor, Donahue worked with combat soldiers who were traumatized by war. Instead of institutionalizing the men, the doctors saw them on an outpatient basis. The doctors had a good success rate in returning these soldiers to their stations. After the war, Donahue worked with Gen. Omar Bradley's office in Washington, DC, to redevelop the Veterans Administration. Donahue then moved to Arkansas, where he helped draft that state's mental health legislation. In 1953, the Oklahoma legislature asked Donahue to develop mental health legislation for the state. In that year, he was appointed Oklahoma's first director of the state's mental health department. In 1961, he became superintendent of Griffin Memorial Hospital. Doctor Donahue's first initiative was to establish a children's ward, as Griffin Memorial was the only state facility with the capabilities to treat children with mental illness. Another of his goals was to establish a vocational rehabilitation center where patients could learn an occupation before leaving the hospital. Donahue also fought for and secured funding to use Griffin Memorial property to house a community health-care center where those with treatable mental illnesses could be seen on an outpatient basis instead of being institutionalized. That community health-care center is now called the Central Oklahoma Community Mental Health Center, and is on the south side of the Griffin Memorial property facing Alameda Street between Southeast Twelfth and Porter Avenues.

The growth of community health-care centers significantly reduced the number of people who were institutionalized across the country. This included the elderly. At one time, Griffin Memorial was a "dumping ground" for elderly citizens who had developed senility and others whose families chose not to (or were not able to) care for them. By the 1960s and 1970s, this was not the case, which further reduced the need for ward buildings that could house patients. At the height of Griffin Memorial Hospital's success as an institution, the hospital owned three farms, where resident farmers and vocational patients tended cows, steers, chickens, hogs, and goats, all of which supplemented the food supply at the institution. There were also vegetable gardens and fruit orchards on the hospital grounds. Today, the only remaining parts of the Griffin Memorial farms are the silos at the corner of Robinson and Southeast Twelfth Avenues adjacent to the old hospital. What was once farmland has been divided into baseball and soccer fields for Norman youth. As with the American Legion Memorial Chapel, the silos stand as a reminder of what was once a significant part of the economic growth of Norman.

One

FROM COLLEGE TO ASYLUM 1890–1914

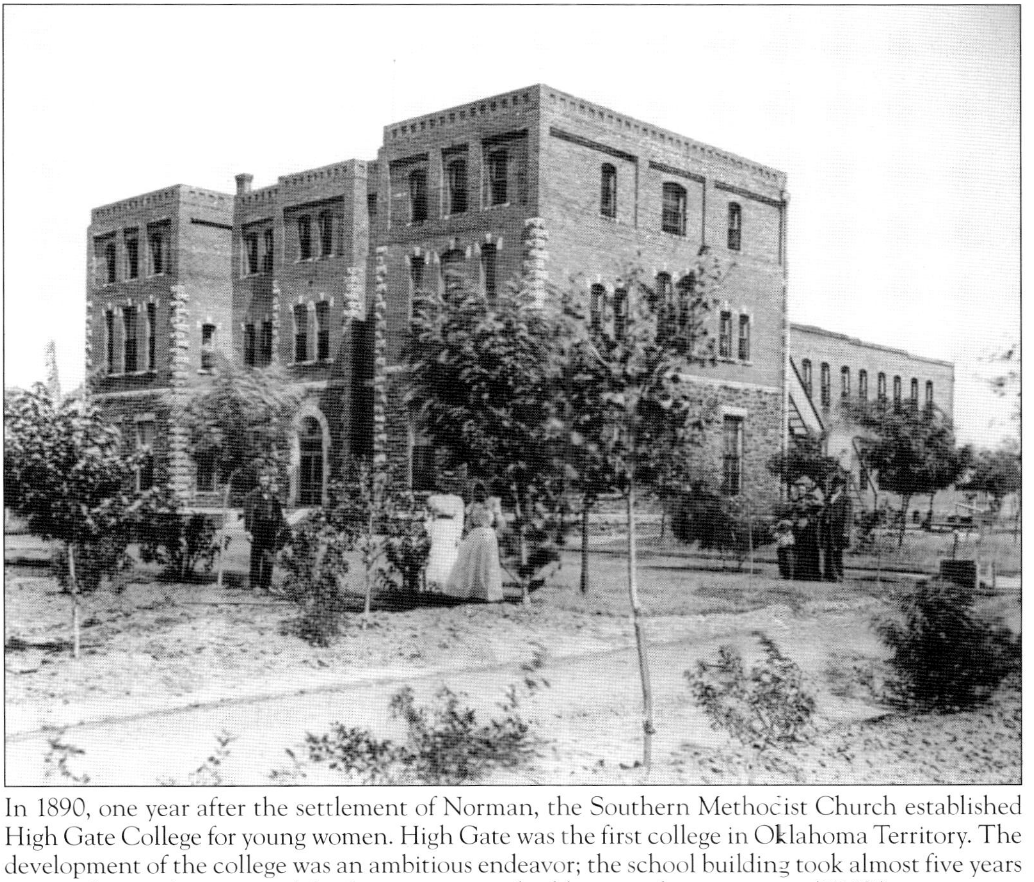

In 1890, one year after the settlement of Norman, the Southern Methodist Church established High Gate College for young women. High Gate was the first college in Oklahoma Territory. The development of the college was an ambitious endeavor; the school building took almost five years to complete and was one of the first permanent buildings in the new town. (OHS.)

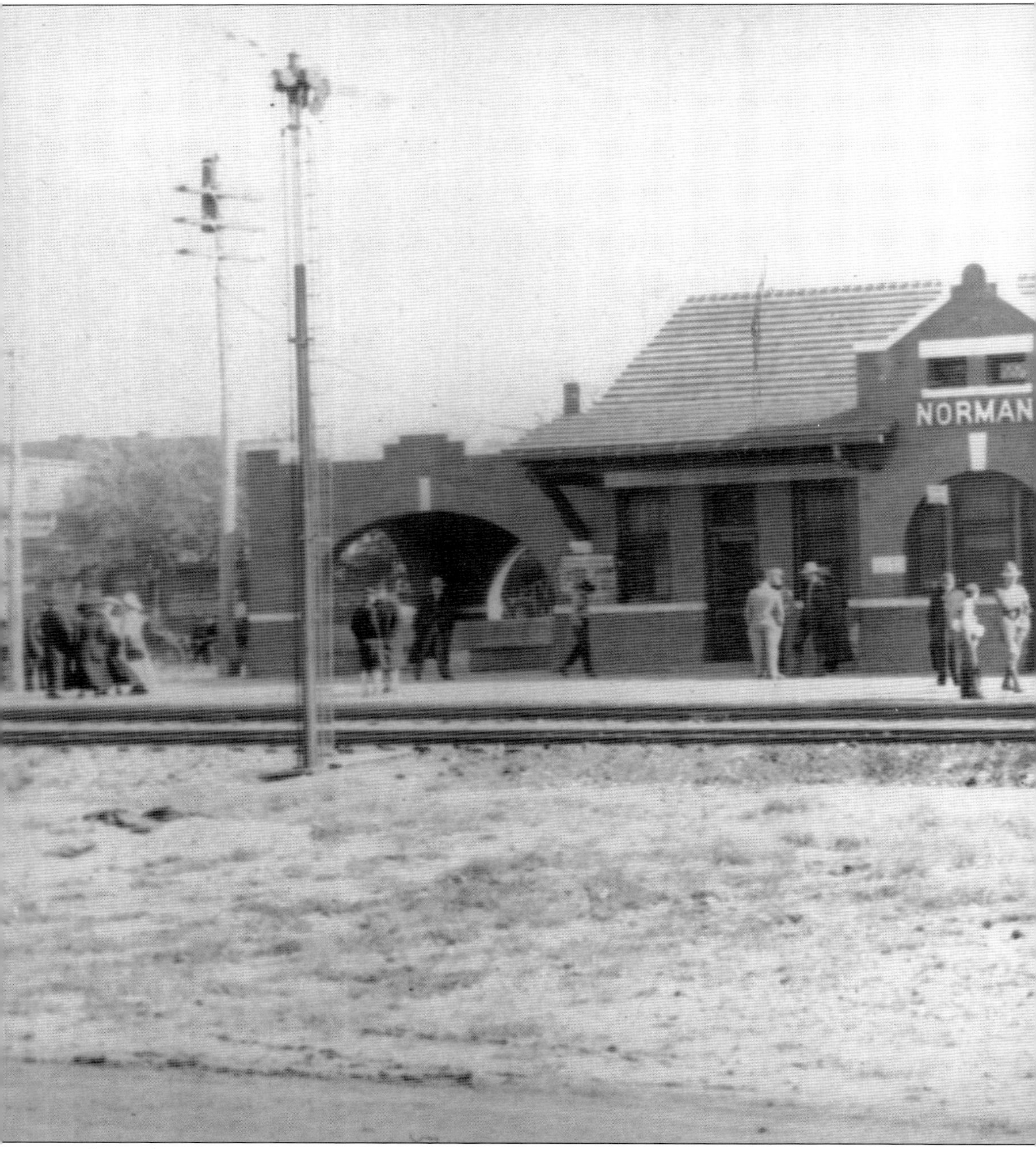

The settlement of Norman began in April 1886, when the Atchison, Topeka & Santa Fe Railway established a depot along its newly laid tracks in preparation for the opening of unassigned lands in central Oklahoma. Train cars full of lumber sat on a siding at the depot waiting for settlers, who marked their land claims in the Land Run of 1889. Once participants in the land run had

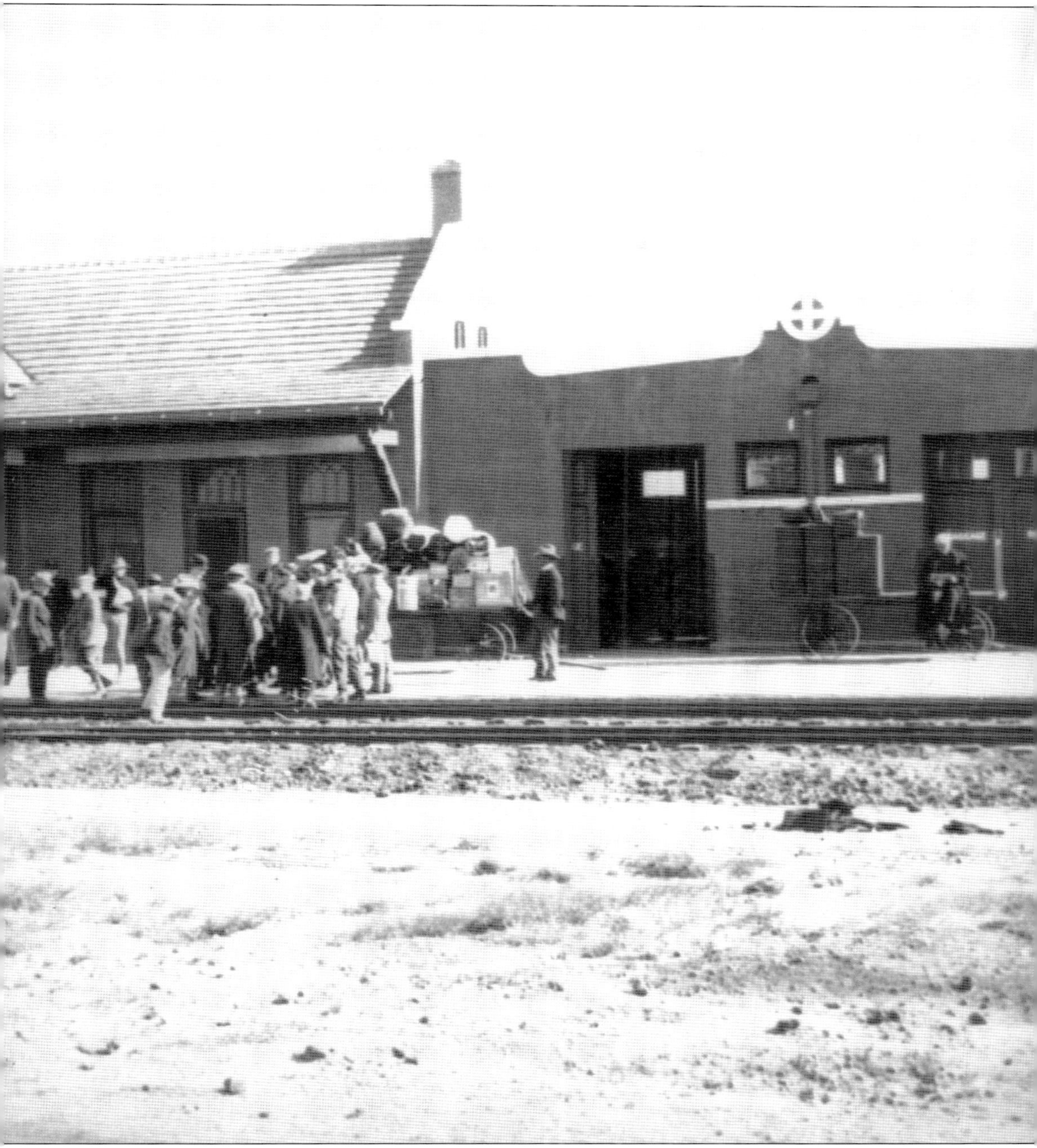

established homesites or businesses, they bought lumber and started to build. In June 1889, two months after the federal government had opened the lands for settlement, Norman's Main Street was lined with a scattering of wood frame buildings. (CCHS.)

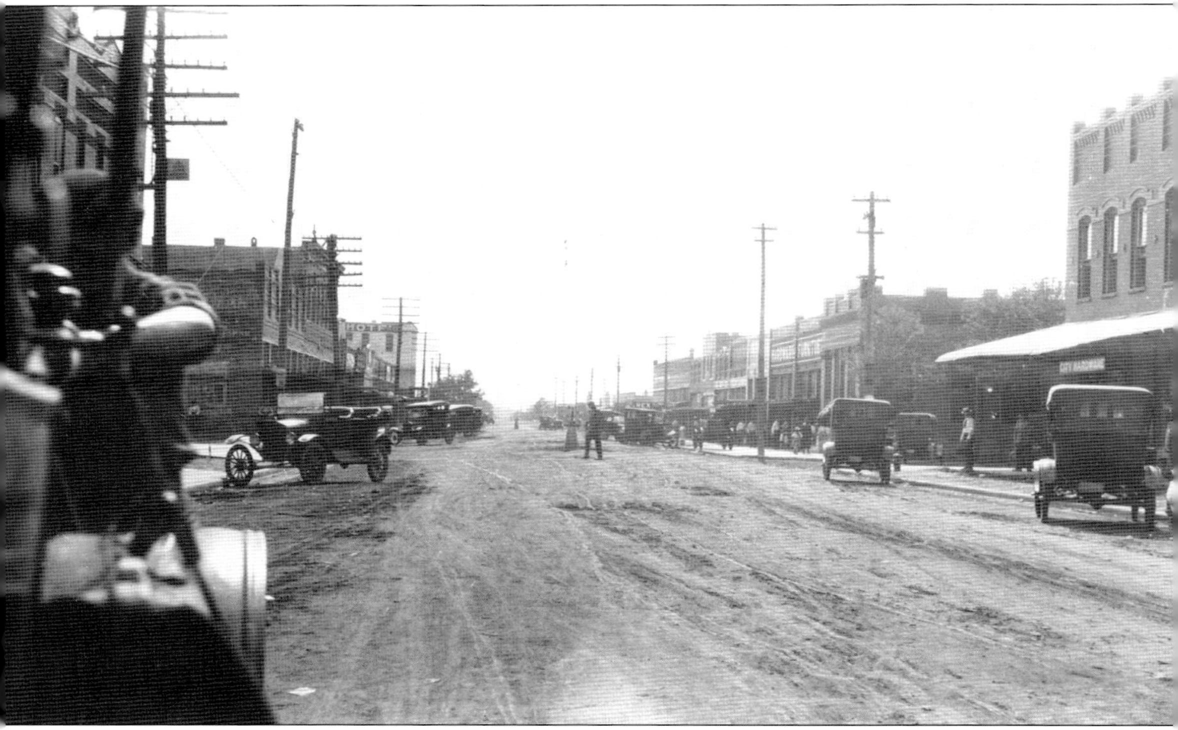

By the early 20th century, Norman had grown into a commercial and agriculture community that served the southern part of the area once called the "Third County." In 1892, the Oklahoma legislature designated Norman as the home of one of the state universities, which later became the University of Oklahoma. In 1893, the legislature chose Norman as the seat of the newly named Cleveland County. The advantage that Norman had over other communities in southern Cleveland County was that the Atchison, Topeka & Santa Fe Railway transported agriculture and livestock to market and in turn brought goods into Norman to be sold at a variety of businesses that lined Main Street. Norman slowly grew into an agricultural and commodity hub and a trade center for the county. New residents found jobs at the University of Oklahoma, the Cleveland County Courthouse, and eventually, High Gate College. (CCHS.)

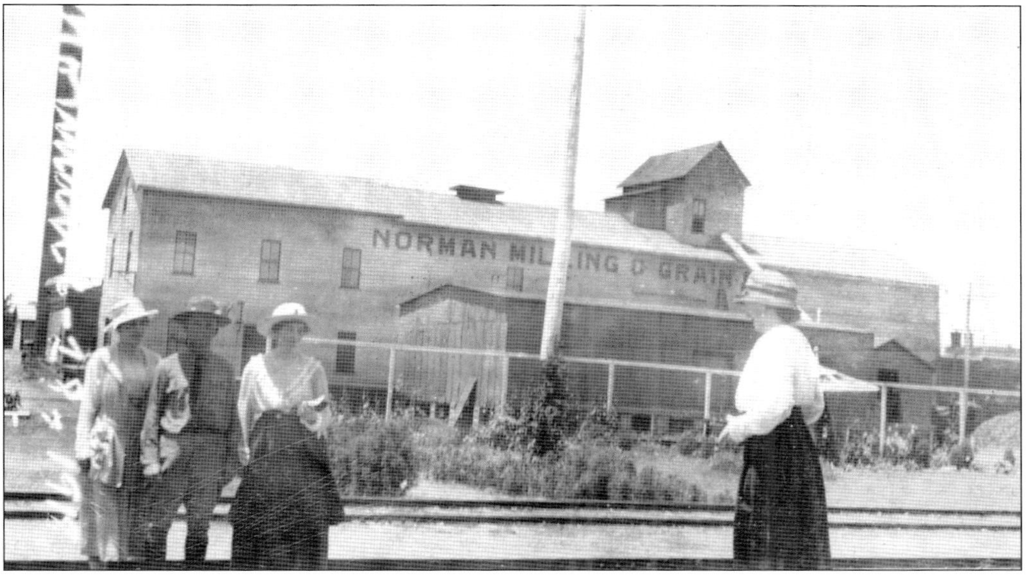

Norman entrepreneurs established businesses that helped the city grow financially. The men who established Norman Milling & Grain in 1891 also gave back to the community. By 1903, the company was providing electricity to the town; its generators ran for three hours after dark. These successful citizens also helped to establish High Gate College. (CCHS.)

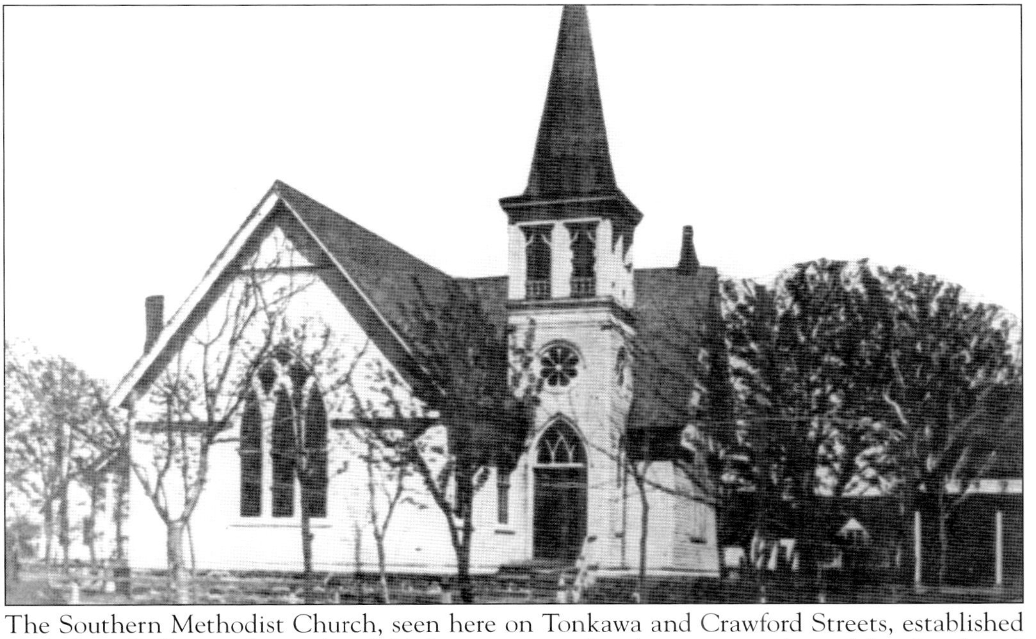

The Southern Methodist Church, seen here on Tonkawa and Crawford Streets, established High Gate College in September 1890. It was a joint effort between members of the church and a citizens' committee made up of Norman's prominent politicians and businessmen. The duty of the committee was to find a suitable building site and secure financial backing. The site was at the end of Main Street on C.J. Bowling's claim. (CCHS.)

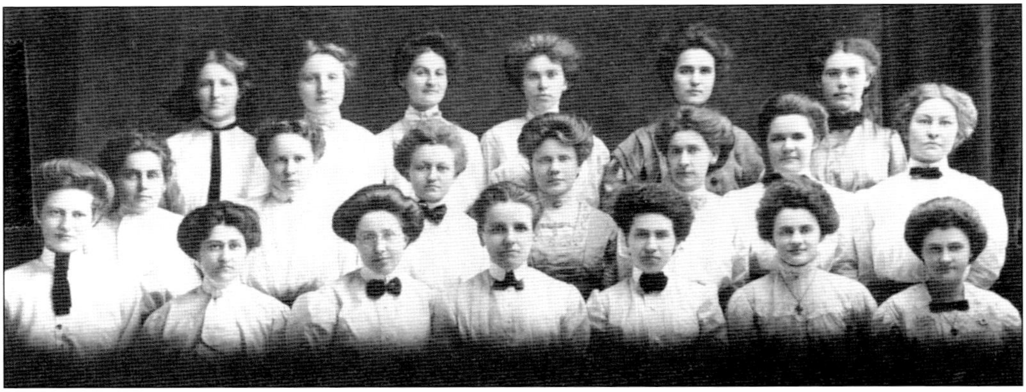

Trustees of the church elected Rev. J.T. Farris as president of High Gate College. The trustees also hired a staff of three teachers. In the first year, 130 women enrolled, and classes were held at the Southern Methodist Church. (CCHS.)

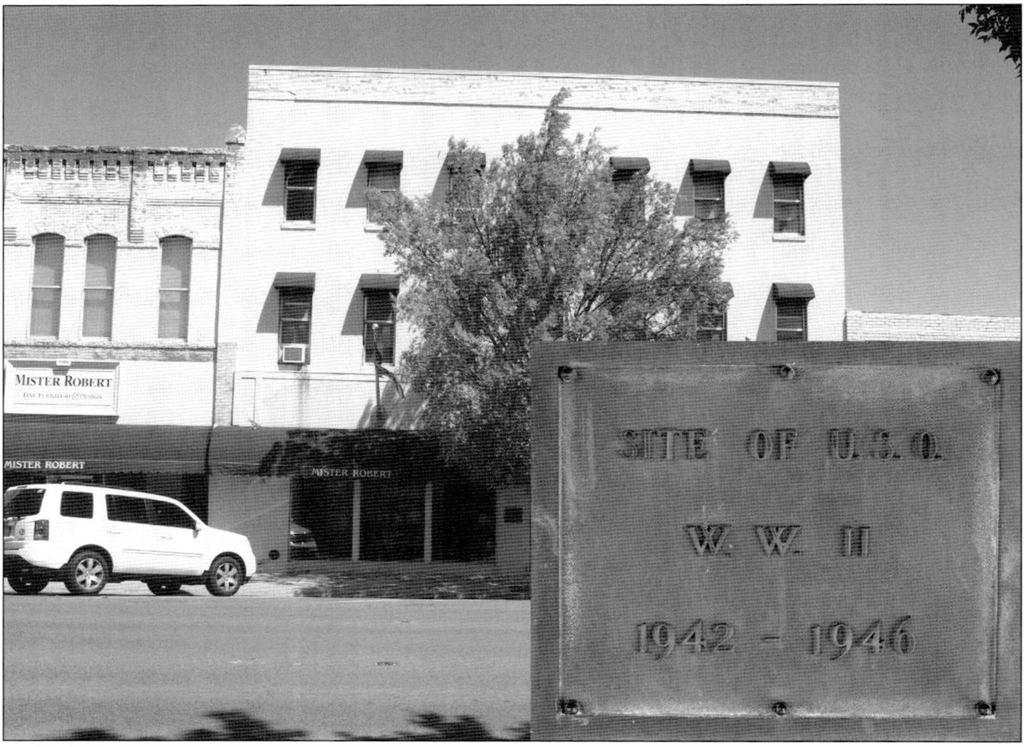

High Gate College graduation ceremonies took place at W.H. Seawell's Opera House at 113 East Main Street (pictured). For the first three years, enrollment increased, but financing was slow in coming to aid with the completion of the administration and classroom building. High Gate College also had competition from the new territorial university located on the second floor of Pryor Adkin's Rock Building at 208 West Main Street. (CCHS.)

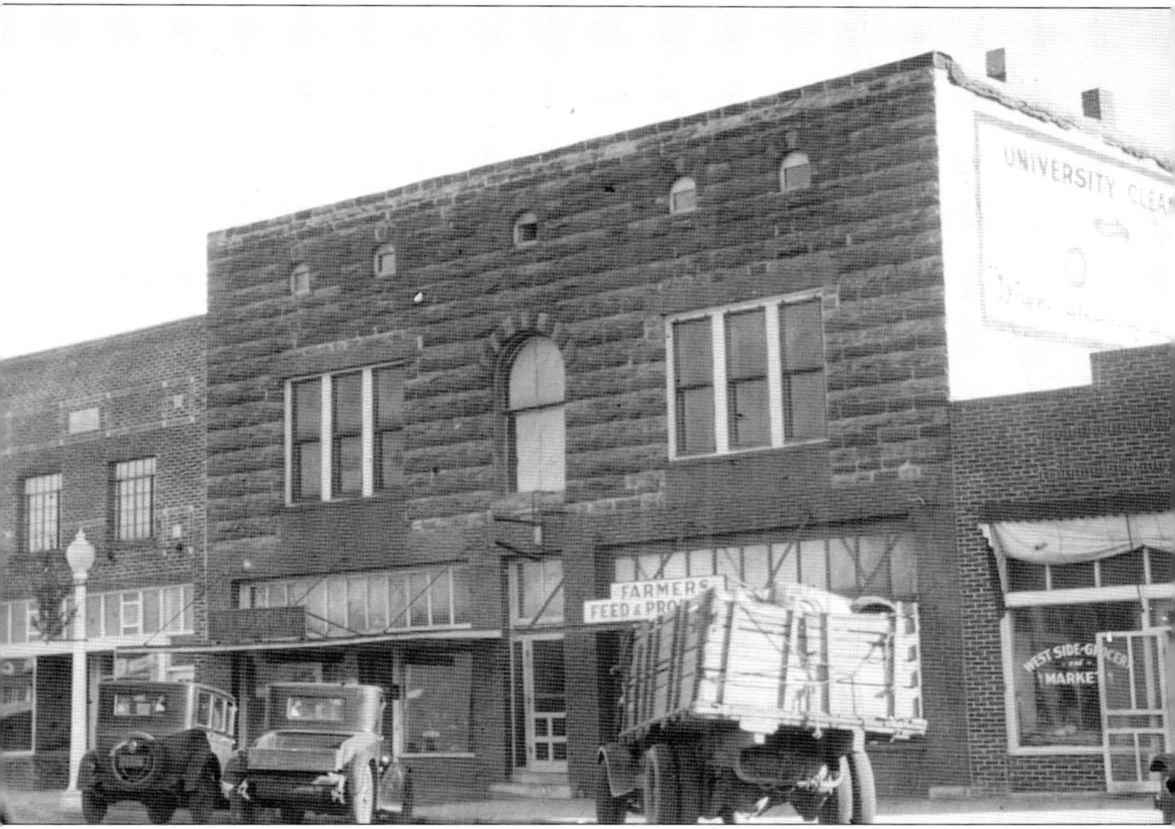

Adkin's Rock Building held the territorial university's first classes when the school opened in 1892. David R. Boyd, the first president of the university, conducted the initial class with a faculty of four for 20 students. Boyd viewed High Gate College, with its 130 students, as being in competition with the University of Oklahoma. Each student at the all-female college paid $3 per month, and High Gate officials held the young women to high moral standards. They were not allowed to participate in recreational activities, especially the popular entertainments of the day. There is little wonder that when the territorial university was established in 1892 with free tuition and no restrictions on student behavior, High Gate started to lose students. Another factor in the decline of the college was the economic depression of 1893, the general lack of interest shown by Norman's civic leaders in High Gate, and the decline of college leadership. High Gate College closed in 1895. (CCHS.)

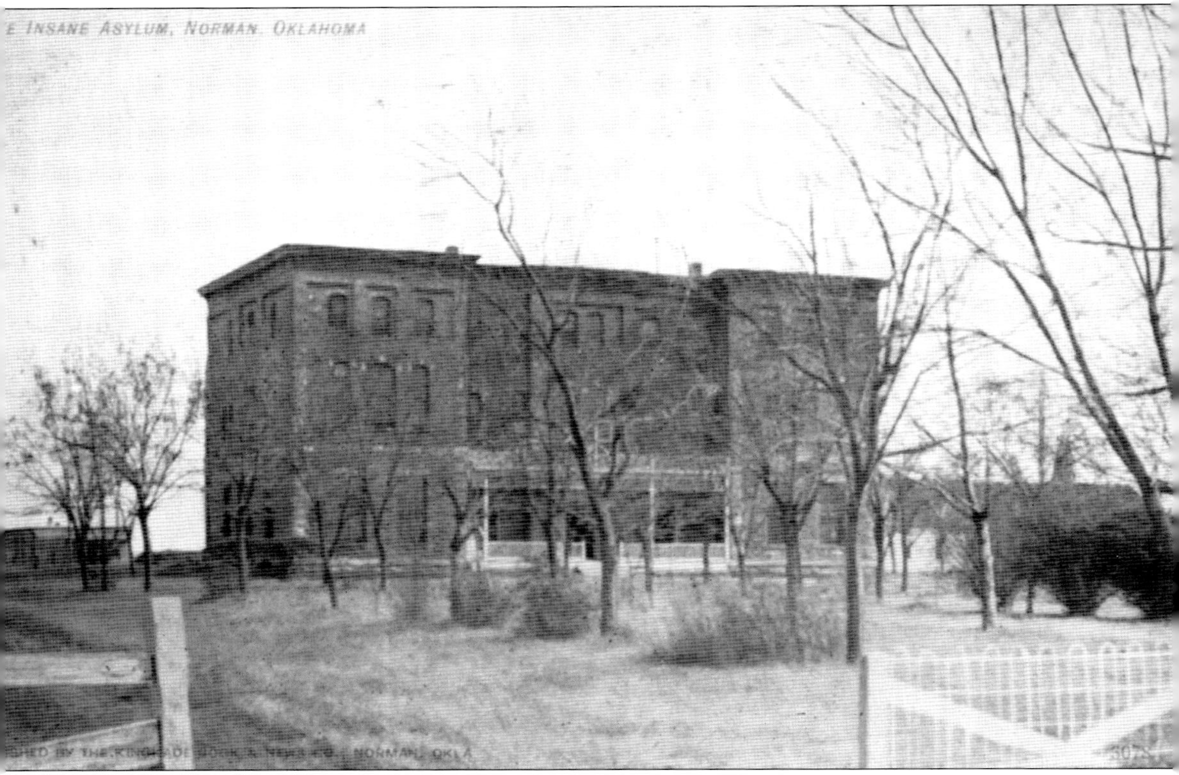

In April 1895, the Oklahoma Sanitarium Company secured a contract from the Oklahoma territorial government for the care of the mentally ill. The company bought the empty and forlorn High Gate College building (pictured) from the City of Norman, and the city donated another 40 acres. (The city had previously bought the land and paid for the building that became High Gate College.) After the building was remodeled and expanded, the Oklahoma Sanitarium opened on June 15, 1895. The *Norman Transcript* reported that a railroad car of "insane people" arrived at the Norman depot and were transported to the sanitarium. Before the sanitarium opened, the territorial government paid $25 per month for the transportation and care of the mentally ill from Oklahoma Territory to Illinois. Upon the opening of the sanitarium, the Oklahoma Sanitarium Company contracted with the territorial government for the care of Oklahoma's mentally ill. This contract benefitted both the territory and the company. (CCHS.)

Dr. John Threadgill was the principle organizer of the incorporated Oklahoma Sanitarium Company. He was born in Wadesboro, North Carolina, in 1847. Threadgill practiced medicine in North Carolina and Texas before he moved to Oklahoma to organize a company to care for the mentally ill. His Oklahoma Sanitarium opened in 1895 with 53 patients. (OHS.)

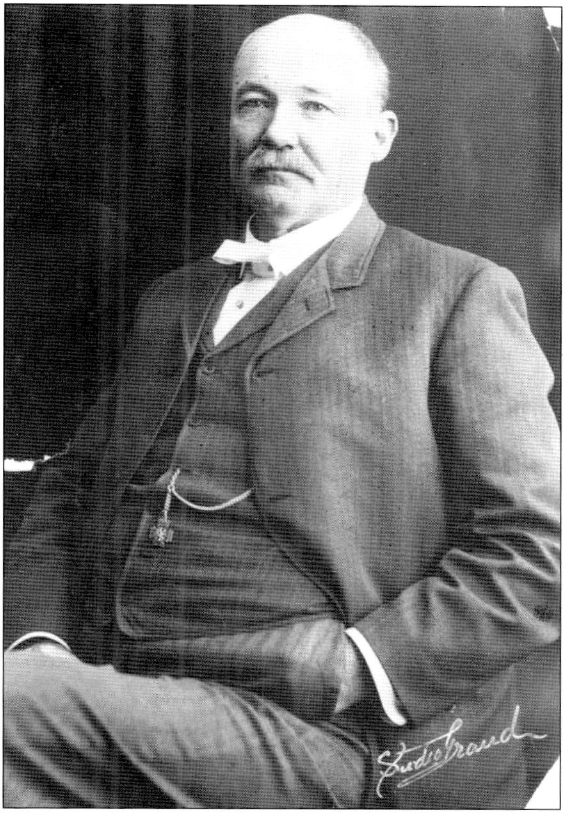

During Dr. Threadgill's tenure as superintendent of the Oklahoma Sanitarium Company from 1895 to 1901, the number of patients increased from 53 in 1895 to 230 in 1899. In 1898, Threadgill secured a contract from the territorial government for $200 per patient per year. Territorial officials who visited the hospital found the sanitarium "neat as a pin" after they toured the facility and met with patients. (OHS.)

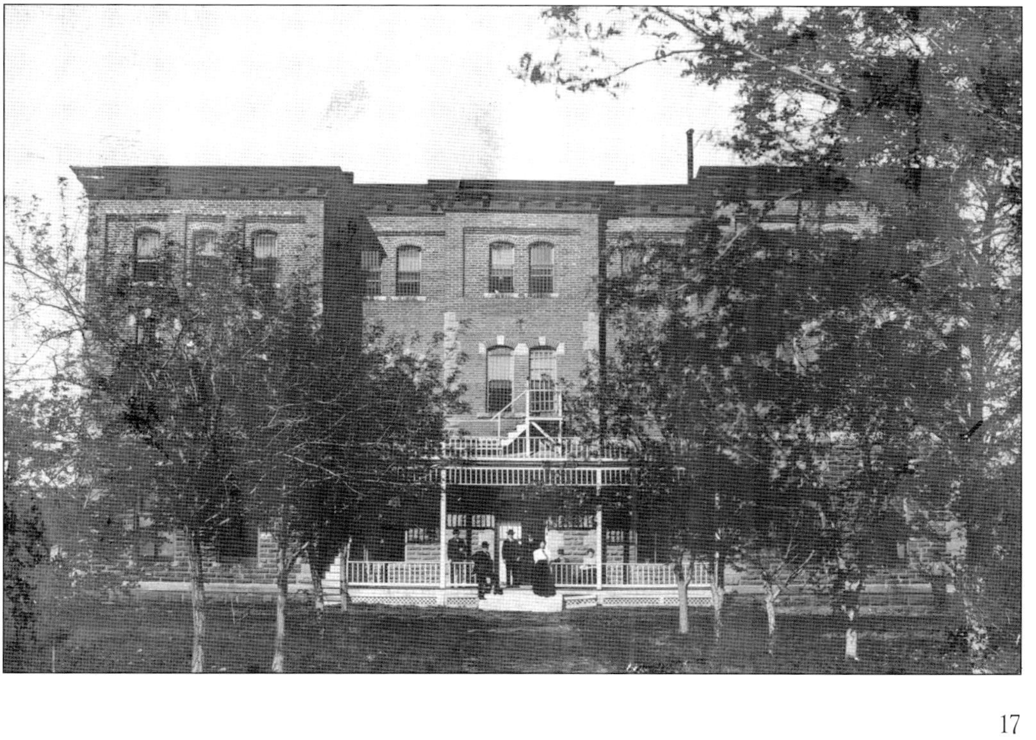

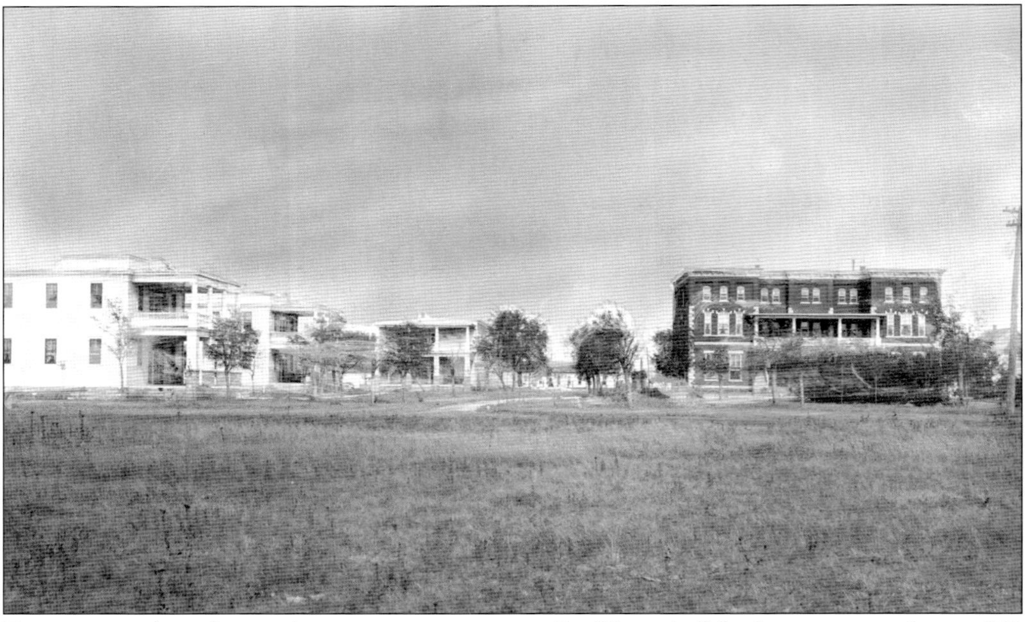

To accommodate the yearly increase in patients, Dr. Threadgill built cottages to house 100 patients. In 1898, wards for men and women were added north of the main building. The old High Gate College building housed a kitchen and dining area in the back and two wards in front. An attendants' ward and laundry were also added. By 1901, additional wards for men and women had been completed. (OHS.)

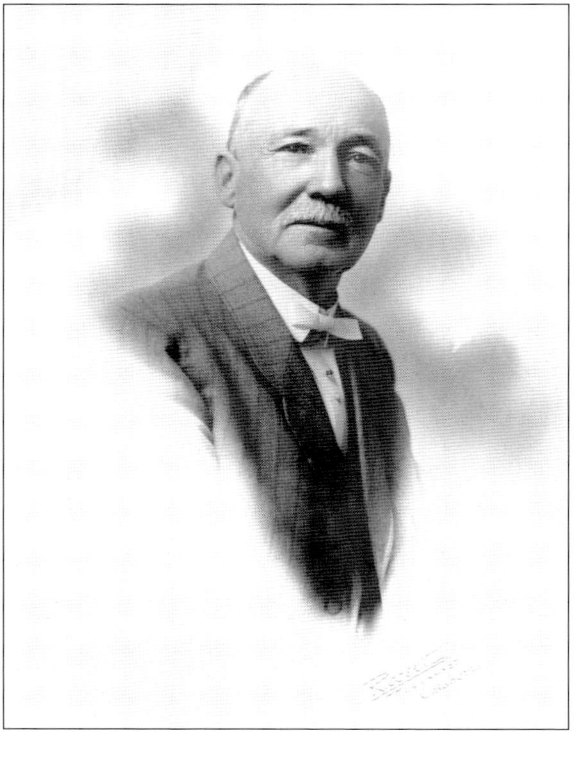

In 1901, Dr. Threadgill sold the Oklahoma Sanitarium Company to a syndicate, which continued to hold the contract with the Oklahoma territorial government for the care of the mentally ill. The governor at the time, William Jenkins, had the authority to offer state contracts; he was also a shareholder in the Oklahoma Sanitarium Company and offered stock options to his friends. Jenkins's political enemies used this issue to unseat the governor. (OHS.)

Pres. William McKinley appointed William Jenkins (pictured) as governor of Oklahoma Territory in 1901. After McKinley was assassinated, Theodore Roosevelt became president. Jenkins's political enemies filed a complaint against him to the US secretary of the interior concerning the Oklahoma Sanitarium Company stock options that Jenkins had offered to his friends. Believing that Jenkins had nefarious stock dealings, Roosevelt relieved Jenkins of his governorship soon after Jenkins assumed office. (OHS.)

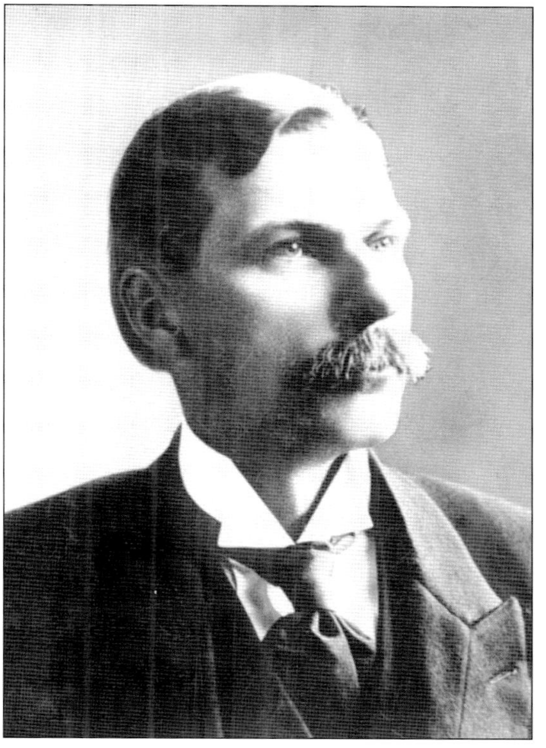

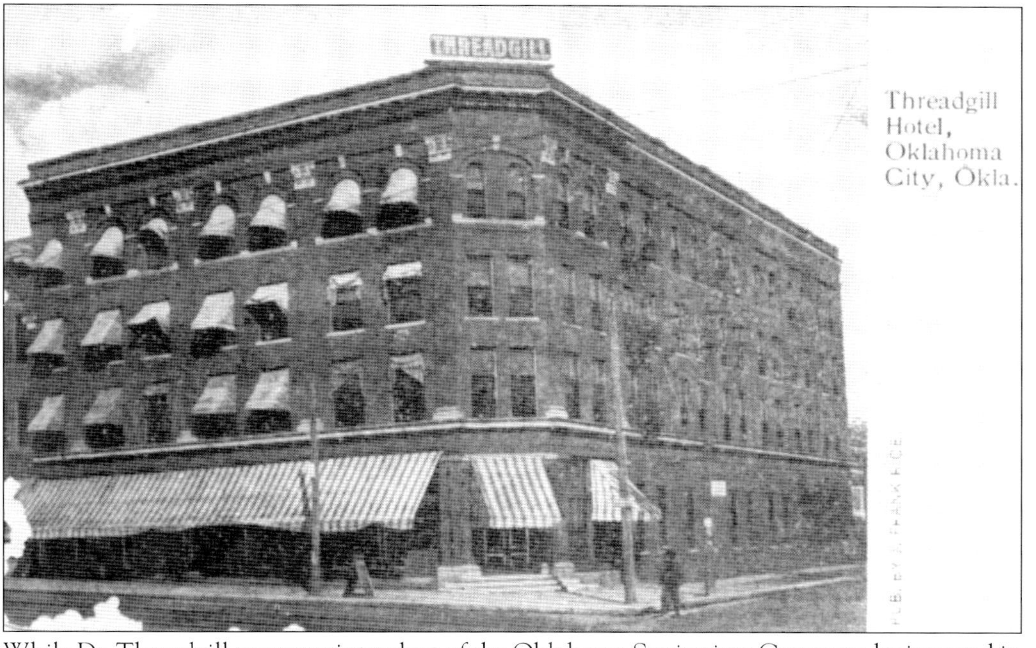

While Dr. Threadgill was superintendent of the Oklahoma Sanitarium Company, he invested in cattle and owned 800 head that he grazed on land outside of Norman. After leaving the Oklahoma Sanitarium Company in 1901, Threadgill moved to Oklahoma City and became a real estate investor. He also established one of the premier hotels in Oklahoma City, the Threadgill. (OHS.)

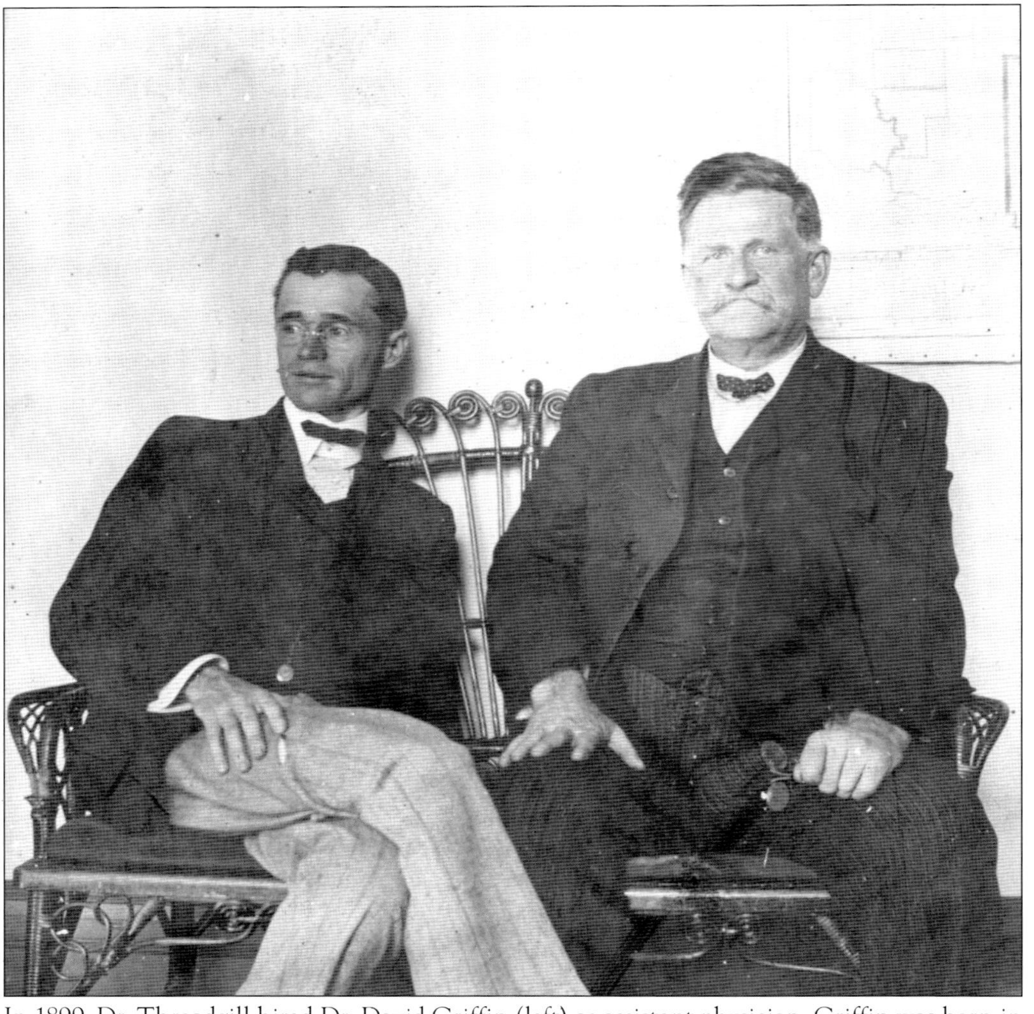

In 1899, Dr. Threadgill hired Dr. David Griffin (left) as assistant physician. Griffin was born in North Carolina in 1875 and graduated from the University of Virginia medical school in 1897. Griffin set up a medical practice and worked in North Carolina until Threadgill offered him a position at the Oklahoma Sanitarium. In his position as assistant physician, Griffin began to implement his theories and treatments for the mentally ill. Griffin believed that many in mental institutions could gain mental wellness and leave the institution. After Threadgill left the Oklahoma Sanitarium Company, Dr. T.C. Clark (right) became superintendent; in that year, there were 325 patients. Upon entering the institution, each patient was assigned an attendant according to the patient's mental difficulties. The territorial legislative report of 1901 gave the Oklahoma Sanitarium a good review, which stated that the grounds were parklike, wards were clean, and patients were well taken care of by the attendants. (OHS.)

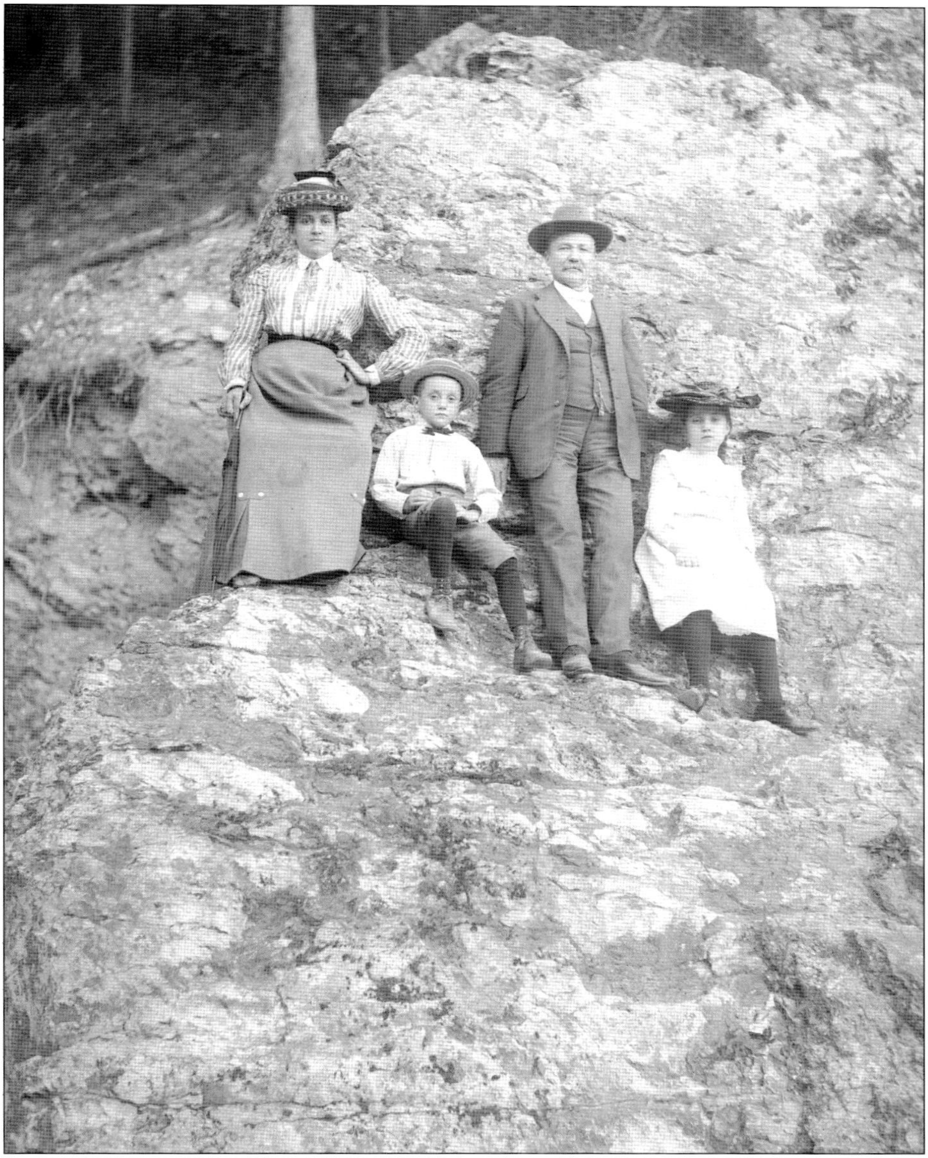

After Dr. Threadgill left the Oklahoma Sanitarium Company, he continued to be involved in the social, economic, and political affairs of Oklahoma City. Threadgill was a Confederate soldier in the Civil War and became commander of the Oklahoma division of the Confederate Veterans Association. When Oklahoma City was part of Oklahoma Territory, Threadgill served as a member of the board of regents of Oklahoma City normal schools and was a four-year member of the Oklahoma City Board of Education, where he served two years as president. Threadgill also organized and incorporated the Commercial National Bank of Oklahoma City. Besides Threadgill's influence in Oklahoma's economic culture, he was interested in politics. In 1903, he was a territorial representative; in 1905, he was a member of the territorial council; and in 1909, he ran for governor of the new state of Oklahoma. Threadgill was married to Frances F. Falwell, and they had three children. Frances was president of the Women's Christian Temperance Union of Oklahoma. (OHS.)

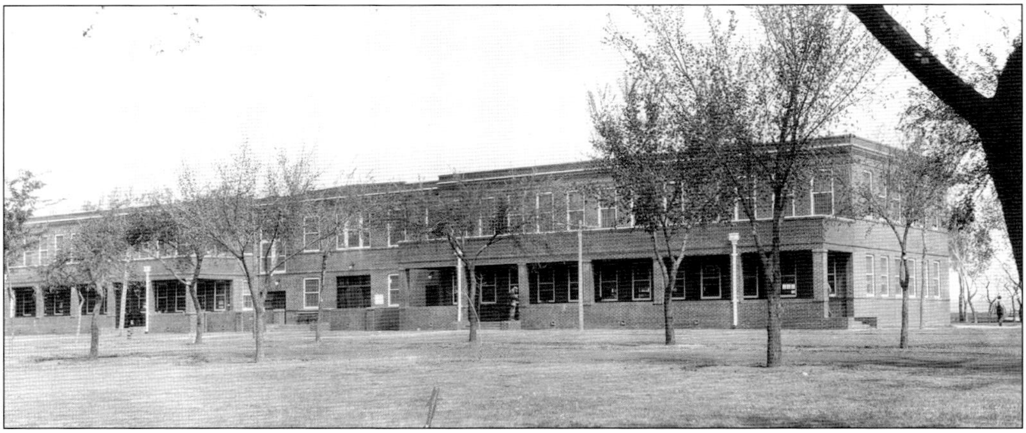

The Oklahoma Sanitarium Company held the first contract for the care of the mentally ill in the territory, but in 1903, the company had competition from the newly established Western State Hospital at Fort Supply (pictured) in western Oklahoma. It was cheaper for the territory to house patients at Western State Hospital, so the legislature made frequent attempts to move patients from the sanitarium in Norman to Western State Hospital. (OHS.)

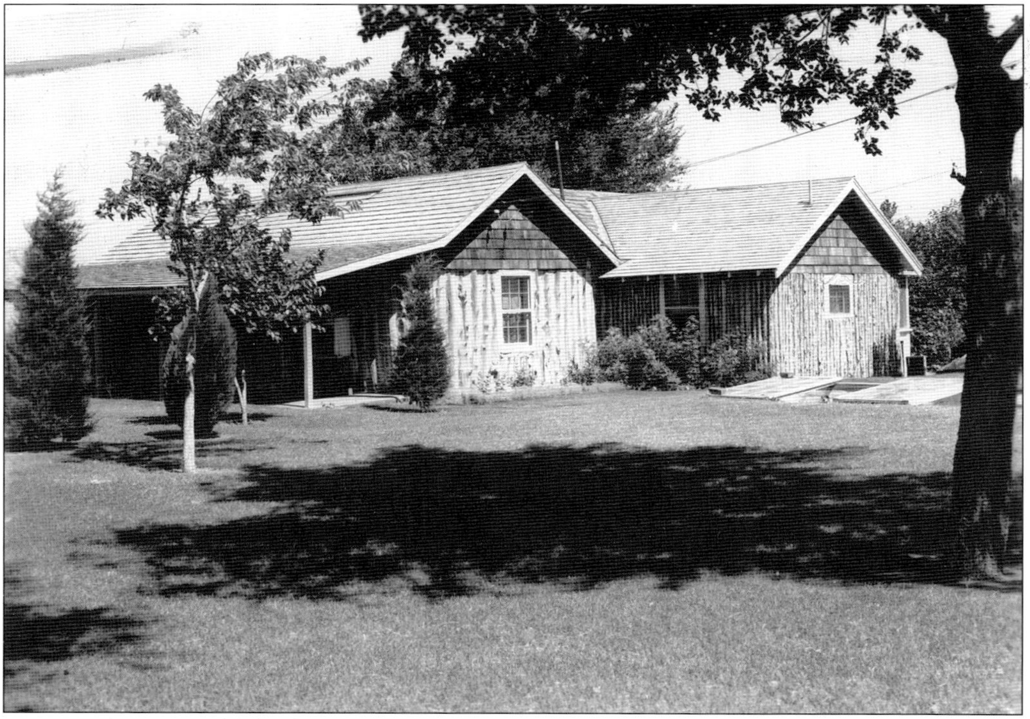

Fort Supply was established in November 1868 as an outpost to support Gen. Phillip Sheridan's winter camp as he fought against the Southern Plains people. Gen. George Armstrong Custer and his Seventh Cavalry also used Fort Supply as an outpost to engage in war against the Cheyenne on the Washita River. (OHS.)

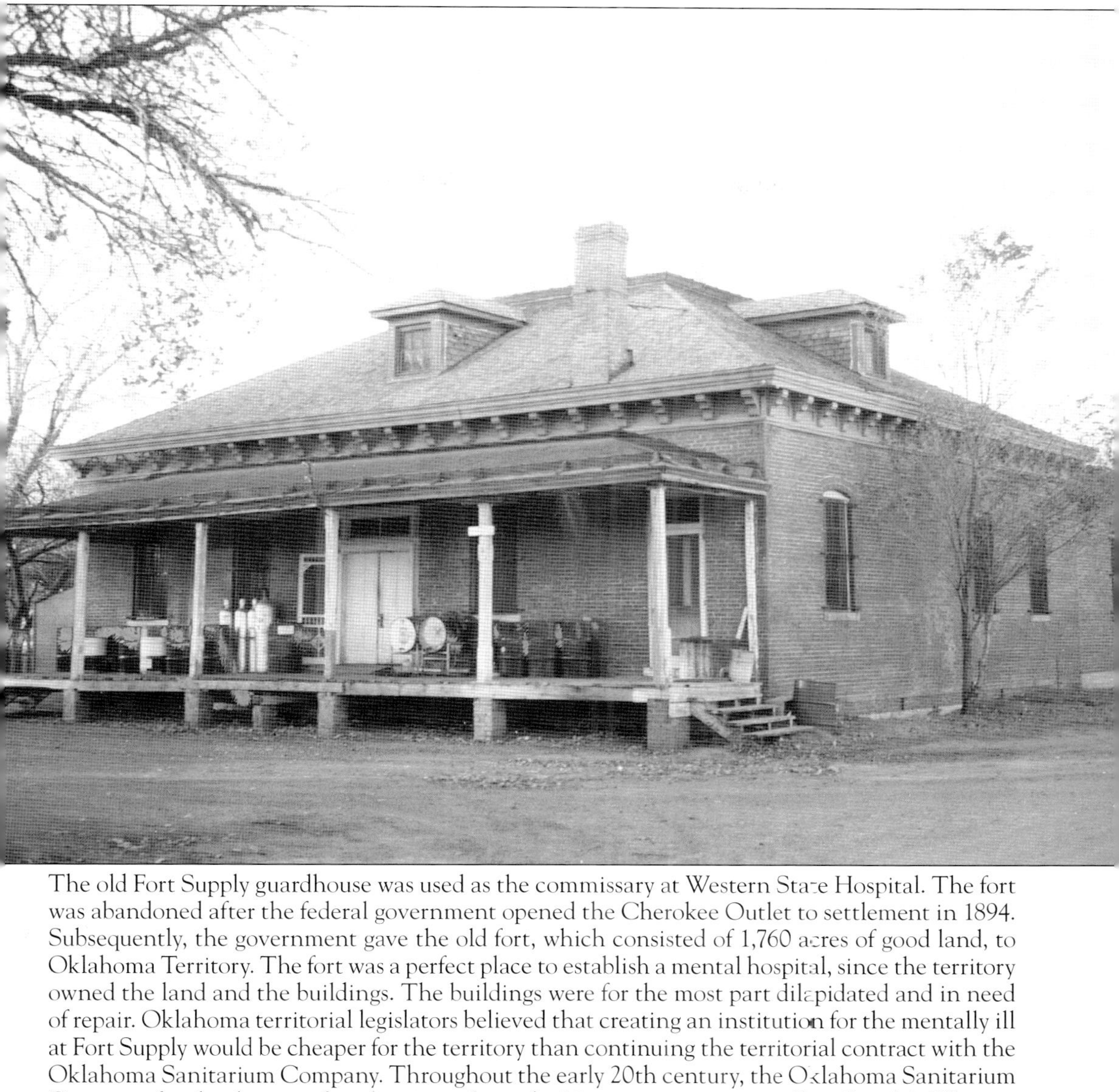

The old Fort Supply guardhouse was used as the commissary at Western State Hospital. The fort was abandoned after the federal government opened the Cherokee Outlet to settlement in 1894. Subsequently, the government gave the old fort, which consisted of 1,760 acres of good land, to Oklahoma Territory. The fort was a perfect place to establish a mental hospital, since the territory owned the land and the buildings. The buildings were for the most part dilapidated and in need of repair. Oklahoma territorial legislators believed that creating an institution for the mentally ill at Fort Supply would be cheaper for the territory than continuing the territorial contract with the Oklahoma Sanitarium Company. Throughout the early 20th century, the Oklahoma Sanitarium Company fought the transfer of patients from the Noman sanitarium to Fort Supply's Western State Hospital. (OHS.)

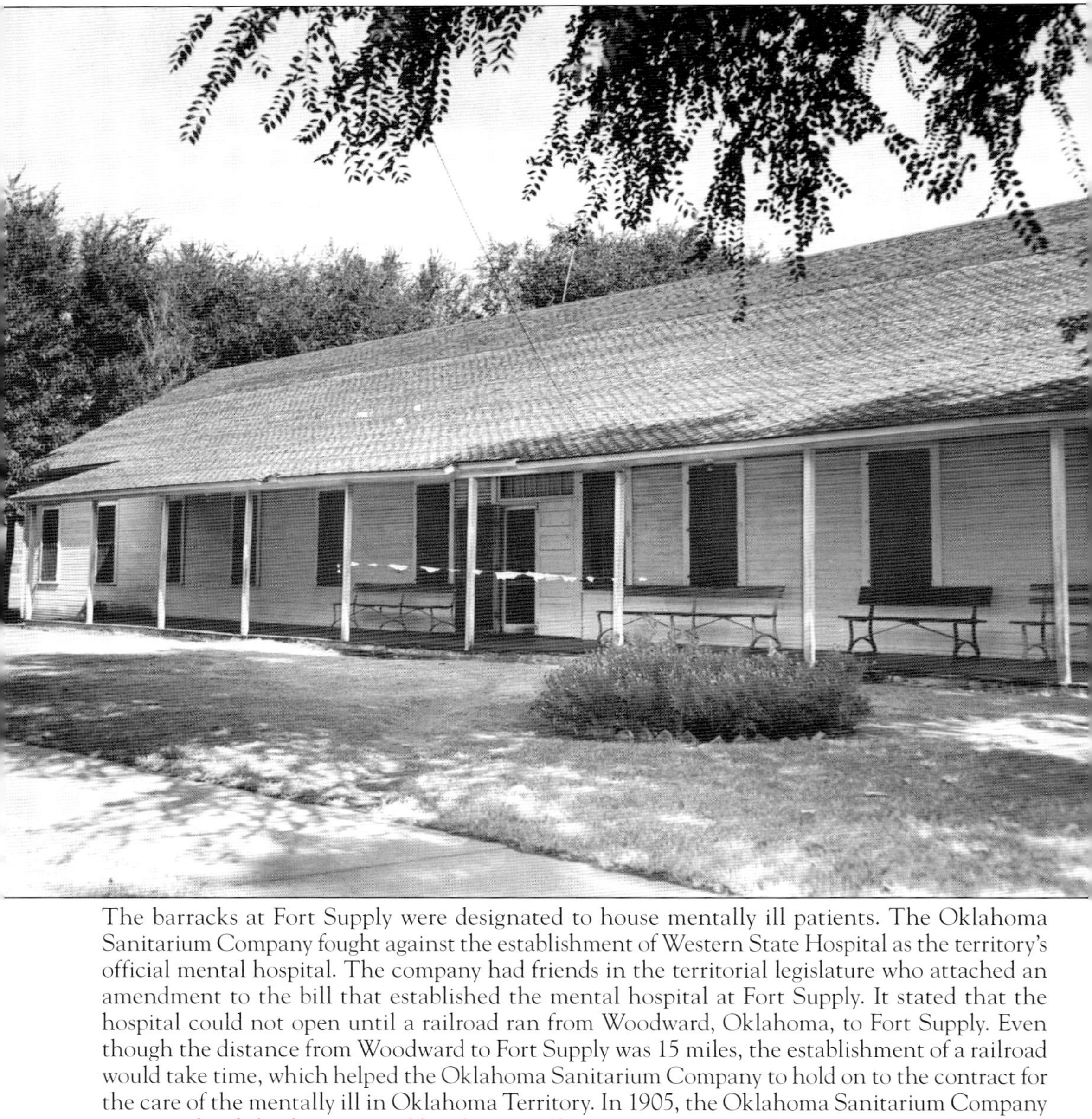

The barracks at Fort Supply were designated to house mentally ill patients. The Oklahoma Sanitarium Company fought against the establishment of Western State Hospital as the territory's official mental hospital. The company had friends in the territorial legislature who attached an amendment to the bill that established the mental hospital at Fort Supply. It stated that the hospital could not open until a railroad ran from Woodward, Oklahoma, to Fort Supply. Even though the distance from Woodward to Fort Supply was 15 miles, the establishment of a railroad would take time, which helped the Oklahoma Sanitarium Company to hold on to the contract for the care of the mentally ill in Oklahoma Territory. In 1905, the Oklahoma Sanitarium Company continued to fight the territorial legislature's efforts to move patients from Norman to Fort Supply. Lawyers for the company filed an injunction on the grounds that the federal government put a moratorium on new construction until after Oklahoma achieved statehood (which occurred in 1907), and Western State Hospital could not build an electrical plant that was needed for asylum operations. (OHS.)

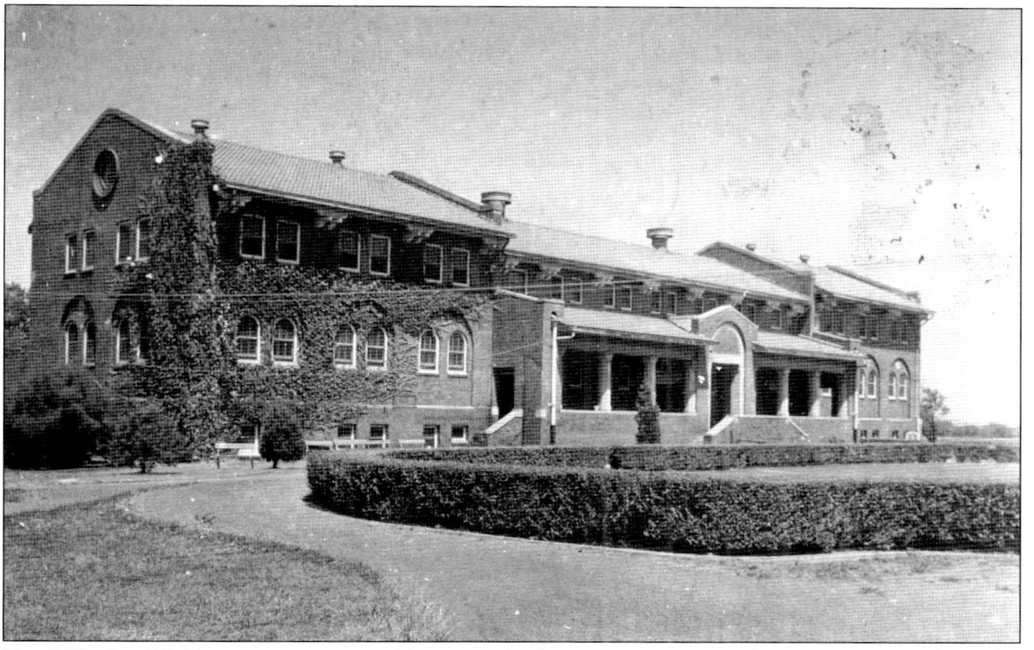

By 1908, the Oklahoma Sanitarium Company had more competition for state money when the legislature passed a bill to establish Eastern State Hospital in Vinita. The legislature appropriated money for 160 acres and $200,000 for buildings. In 1909, the Oklahoma Asylum Board recommended $500,000 for taking care of the mentally ill in the eastern part of the new state. (OHS.)

After the establishment of state asylums in western and eastern Oklahoma (pictured), legislators and newspaper editors believed it was only a matter of time before the unprofitable Oklahoma Sanitarium Company would be bought by the state to serve central Oklahoma. Before that happened, however, Kate Barnard, commissioner of charities and corrections in Oklahoma's first legislature, toured the asylums and made a scathing report to the state. (OHS.)

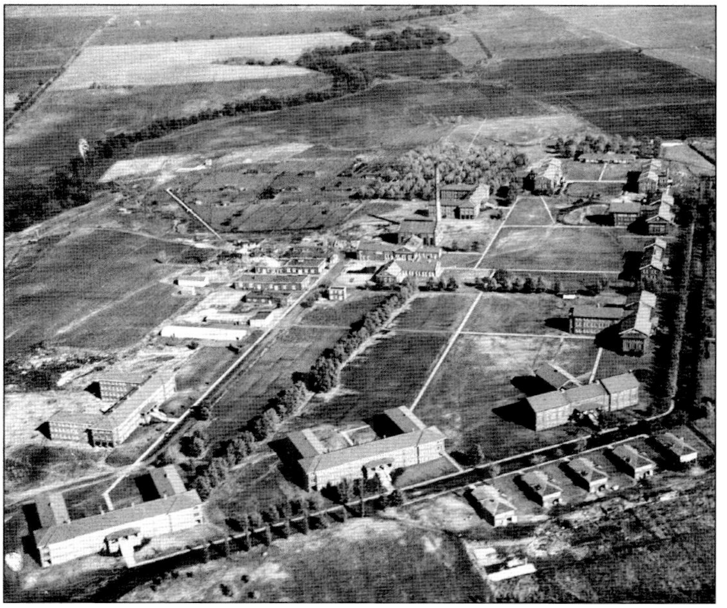

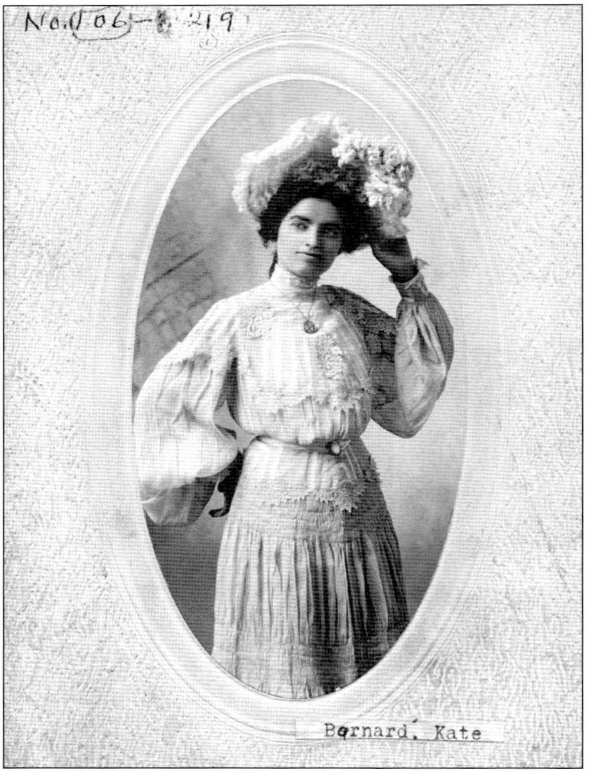

Part of the responsibilities assigned to Kate Barnard, commissioner of charities and corrections in Oklahoma's first legislature, included the inspection of state institutions and institutions that held state contracts. Barnard spent four days inspecting the Oklahoma Sanitarium in Norman in 1909. Her report condemned the management for their incompetent supervision of inmates; she claimed management only cared about private stockholders. (OHS.)

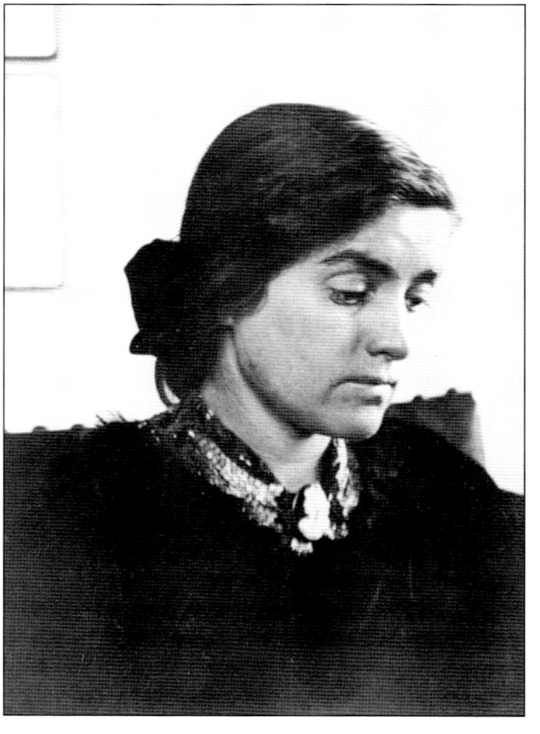

Barnard's report to Gov. Charles N. Haskell also cited brutality toward patients from attendants, intermingling of white and black patients, and extreme overcrowding. Barnard also claimed that the sanitarium's high death rate (81 patients died in 1909) could be avoided with proper nutrition. Barnard's report demanded remedies or else she would take the Oklahoma Sanitarium Company to court. (CCHS.)

One of the demands made by Barnard in her 1909 inspection report was that Oklahoma Sanitarium superintendent A.H. Clark be removed. Dr. David Griffin (pictured) took Clark's place as superintendent in 1910. Barnard recommended that the asylum purchase 2,500 blankets, 50 rocking chairs, and heaters for each room. She also wanted the rooms painted and windows installed in the windowless halls. Barnard suggested the purchase of fruits and vegetables to augment healthier diets, especially for the older patients. (OHS.)

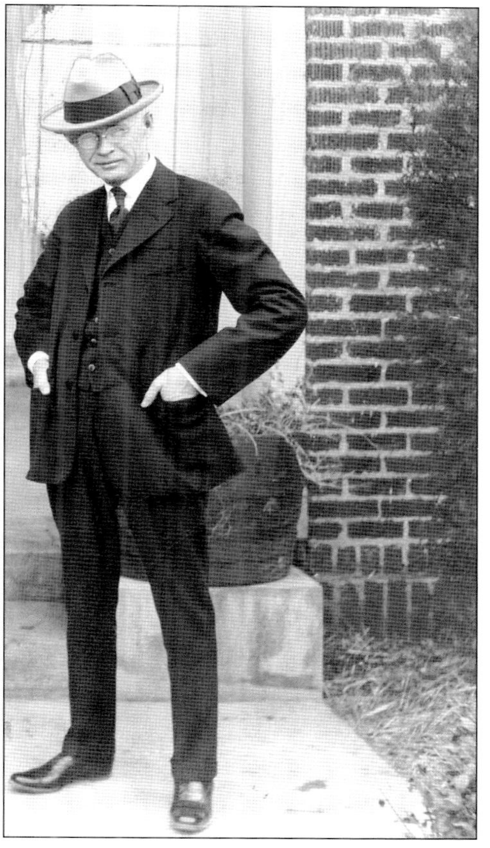

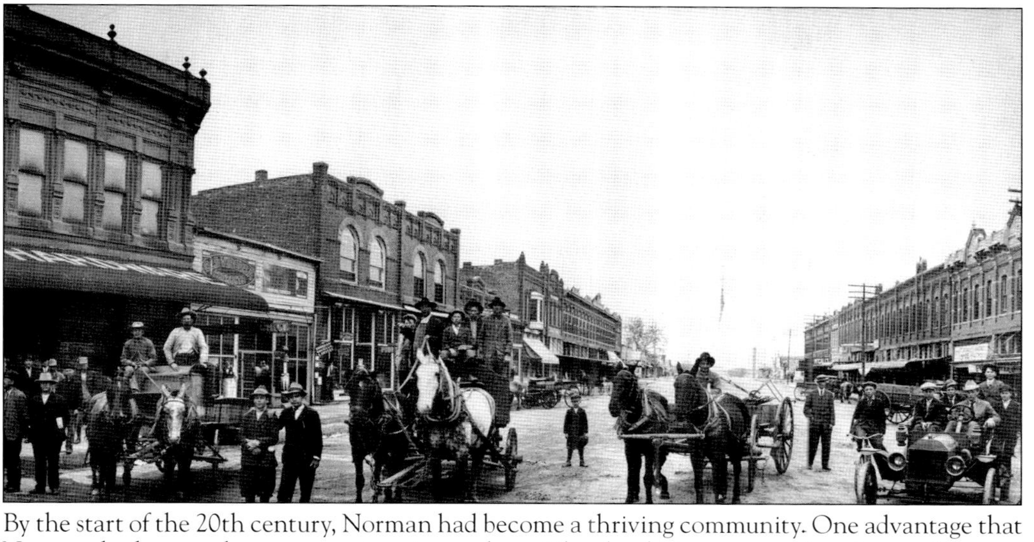

By the start of the 20th century, Norman had become a thriving community. One advantage that Norman had over other communities in southern Cleveland County was that the employment offered by Norman's commodity center and the University of Oklahoma, Cleveland County Courthouse, and the Oklahoma Sanitarium Company enhanced the town's ability to grow, and it eventually became the state's third-largest city. (CCHS.)

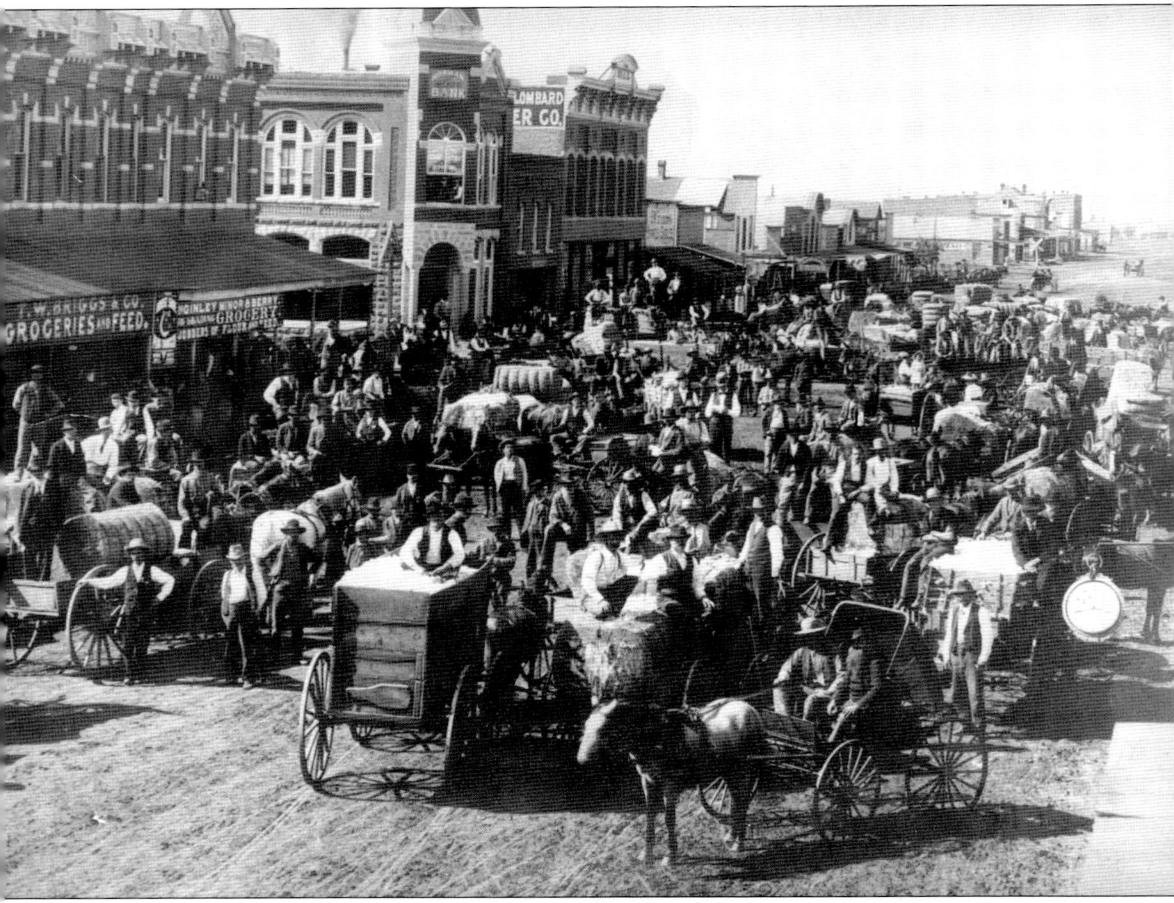

Norman emerged as a prosperous agricultural community alongside the growth of the Oklahoma Sanitarium. After Oklahoma became a state in 1907, the sanitarium found it difficult to compete for state contracts. Consequently, in 1915, the state bought the Oklahoma Sanitarium Company and established Central State Hospital. (CCHS.)

Two

Growth of an Institution 1915–1939

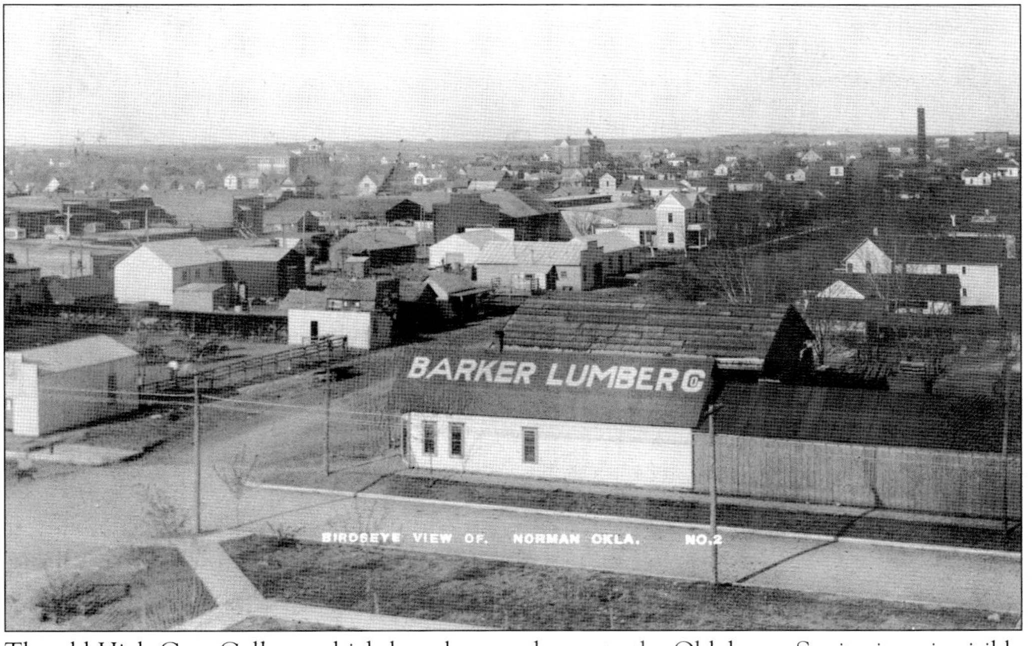

The old High Gate College, which later became home to the Oklahoma Sanitarium, is visible in the upper right of this photograph. In 1915, the State of Oklahoma bought the Oklahoma Sanitarium Company and renamed the institution Central State Hospital. Throughout the early 20th century, hospital superintendent Dr. David Griffin lobbied for state appropriations for new ward buildings, and initiated new modern treatments for the mentally ill. (CCHS.)

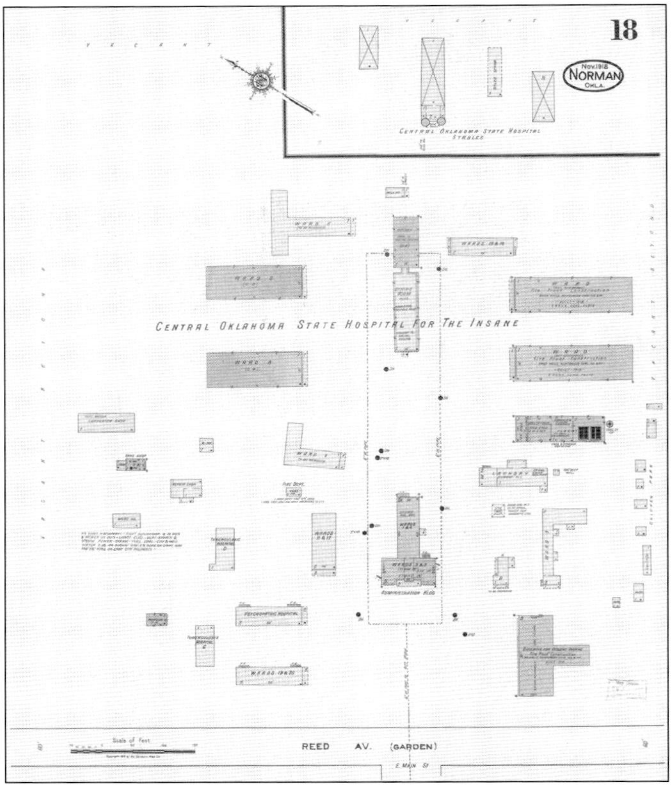

In 1915, the fifth Oklahoma legislature adopted a resolution for the purchase of the Oklahoma Sanitarium Company. The $100,000 purchase included several tracts of land as well as sanitarium buildings and equipment, as seen on this 1914 Sanborn insurance map. Acquiring the sanitarium saved the state money, because the contract with the Oklahoma Sanitarium Company was more costly than the appropriations granted to the Western and Eastern State Hospitals. (CCHS.)

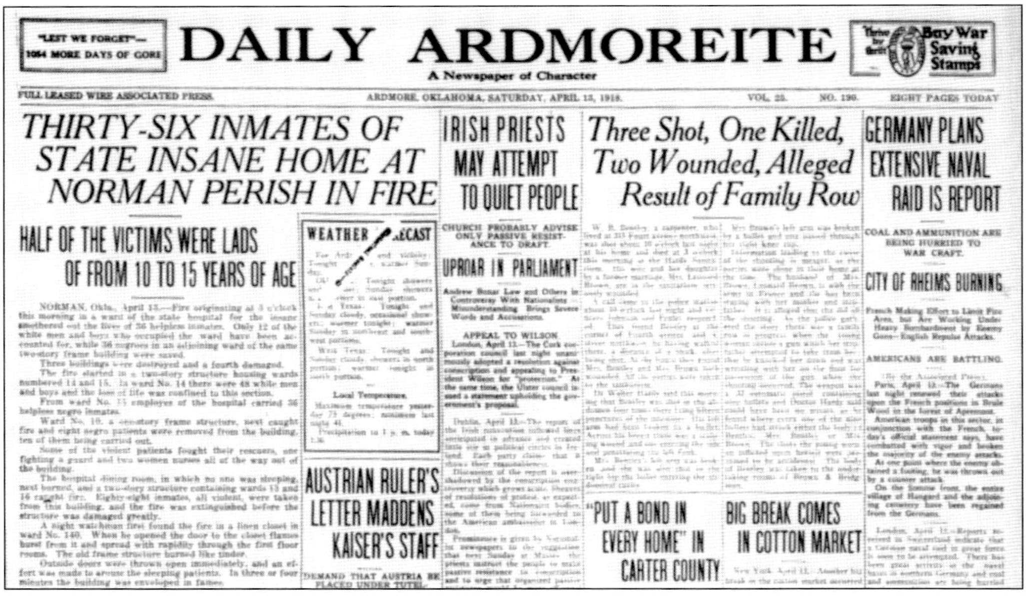

"LEST WE FORGET"—1054 MORE DAYS OF GORE

DAILY ARDMOREITE

A Newspaper of Character

Thrive by thrift — Buy War Savings Stamps

FULL LEASED WIRE ASSOCIATED PRESS. ARDMORE, OKLAHOMA, SATURDAY, APRIL 13, 1918. VOL. 25. NO. 190. EIGHT PAGES TODAY

THIRTY-SIX INMATES OF STATE INSANE HOME AT NORMAN PERISH IN FIRE

HALF OF THE VICTIMS WERE LADS OF FROM 10 TO 15 YEARS OF AGE

NORMAN, Okla., April 13.—Fire originating at 3 o'clock this morning in a ward of the state hospital for the insane smothered out the lives of 36 helpless inmates. Only 12 of the white men and boys who occupied the ward have been accounted for, while 36 negroes in an adjoining ward of the same two-story frame building were saved.

Three buildings were destroyed and a fourth damaged.

The fire started in a two-story structure housing wards numbered 14 and 15. In ward No. 14 there were 48 white men and boys and the loss of life was confined to this section.

From ward No. 15 employes of the hospital carried 36 helpless negro inmates.

Ward No. 10, a one-story frame structure, next caught fire and eight negro patients were removed from the building, ten of them being carried out.

Some of the violent patients fought their rescuers, one fighting a guard and two women nurses all of the way out of the building.

The hospital dining room, in which no one was sleeping, next burned, and a two-story structure containing wards 13 and 16 caught fire. Eighty-eight inmates, all violent, were taken from this building, and the fire was extinguished before the structure was damaged greatly.

A night watchman first found the fire in a linen closet in ward No. 140. When he opened the door to the closet flames burst from it and spread with rapidity through the first floor rooms. The old frame structure burned like tinder.

Outside doors were thrown open immediately, and an effort was made to arouse the sleeping patients. In three or four minutes the building was enveloped in flames.

WEATHER FORECAST

AUSTRIAN RULER'S LETTER MADDENS KAISER'S STAFF

IRISH PRIESTS MAY ATTEMPT TO QUIET PEOPLE

CHURCH PROBABLY ADVISE ONLY PASSIVE RESISTANCE TO DRAFT.

UPROAR IN PARLIAMENT

APPEAL TO WILSON

Three Shot, One Killed, Two Wounded, Alleged Result of Family Row

"PUT A BOND IN EVERY HOME" IN CARTER COUNTY

BIG BREAK COMES IN COTTON MARKET

GERMANY PLANS EXTENSIVE NAVAL RAID IS REPORT

COAL AND AMMUNITION ARE BEING HURRIED TO WAR CRAFT.

CITY OF RHEIMS BURNING

AMERICANS ARE BATTLING.

At 3:00 a.m. on April 13, 1918, the night watchman at Central State Hospital, L.T. Hawes, discovered a fire in the linen closet of ward 14. Hawes hurried to unlock the doors and called an alarm with the steam whistle. The asylum's fire crew, nurses, and staff immediately started to evacuate the ward, which housed 48 men and boys; however, 40 of them perished in the fire. (CCHS.)

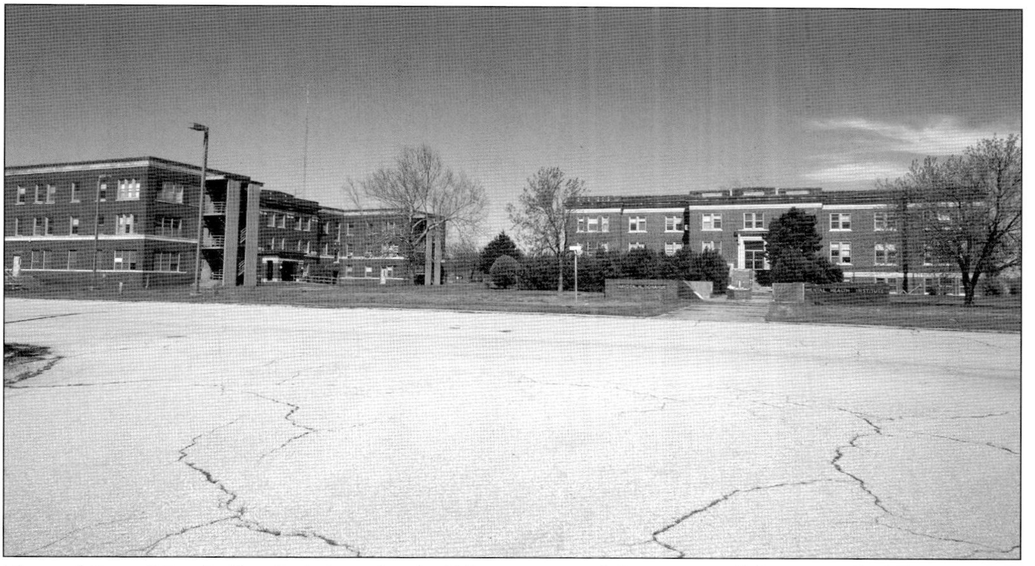

Central State Hospital's administration building occupied the center of the grounds. The women's wards (pictured) were to the north, and the men's wards were to the south. The 40 men and young boys who died in the April 1918 fire were from ward 14. The upper floor, ward 15, housed Black patients, who survived the fire. At the time of the 1920 census, there were 1,100 patients at Central State, and 299 of them were Black. (CCHS.)

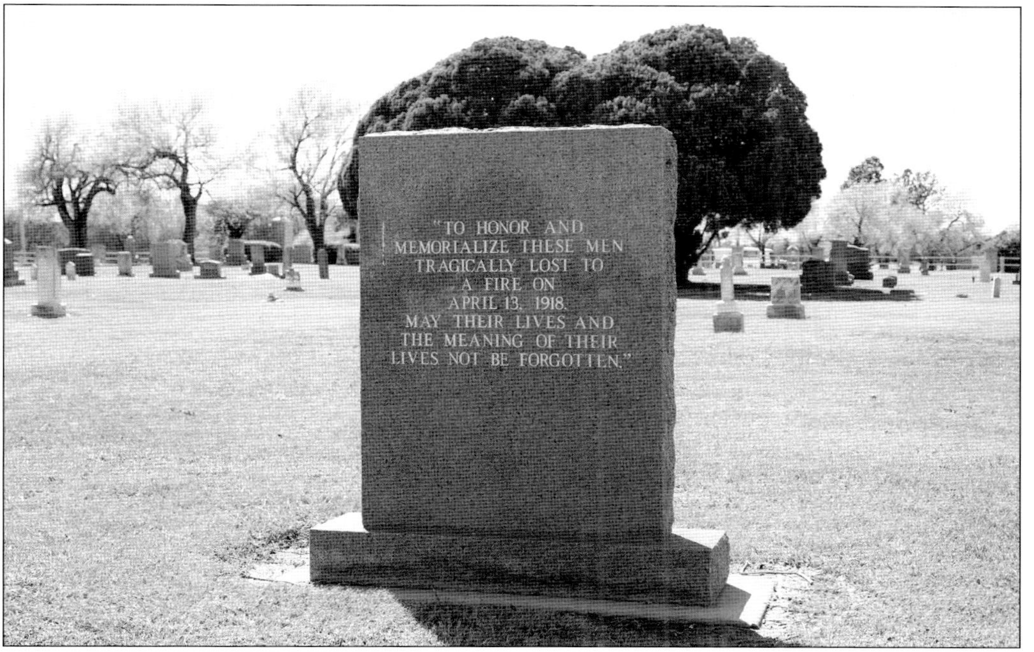
"TO HONOR AND
MEMORIALIZE THESE MEN
TRAGICALLY LOST TO
A FIRE ON
APRIL 13, 1918.
MAY THEIR LIVES AND
THE MEANING OF THEIR
LIVES NOT BE FORGOTTEN."

The 40 men and boys who perished in the April 1918 fire at Central State Hospital were laid to rest in pine boxes in a mass grave at the Independent Order of Odd Fellows Cemetery in Norman. For 100 years, the location of the grave site was unknown. Using new technology, the Oklahoma Archeological Survey found the site in 2015. In April 2015, citizens of Norman dedicated a marker recognizing those who lost their lives in the fire. (CCHS.)

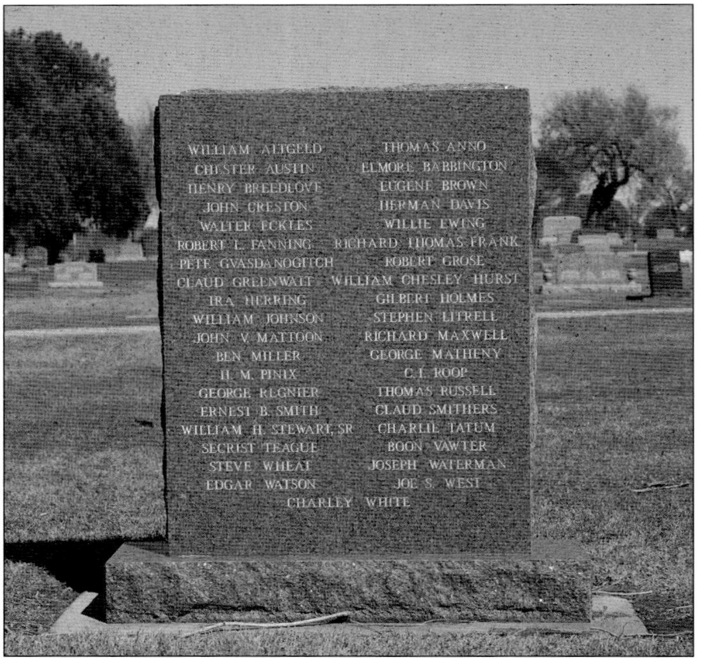
WILLIAM ALTGELD
THOMAS ANNO
CHESTER AUSTIN
ELMORE BARBINGTON
HENRY BREEDLOVE
EUGENE BROWN
JOHN CRESTON
HERMAN DAVIS
WALTER ECKLES
WILLIE EWING
ROBERT L. FANNING
RICHARD THOMAS FRANK
PETE GVASDANOGITCH
ROBERT GROSE
CLAUD GREENWALT
WILLIAM CHESLEY HURST
IRA HERRING
GILBERT HOLMES
WILLIAM JOHNSON
STEPHEN LITRELL
JOHN V. MATTOON
RICHARD MAXWELL
BEN MILLER
GEORGE MATHENY
H. M. PINIX
C.I. ROOP
GEORGE REGNIER
THOMAS RUSSELL
ERNEST B. SMITH
CLAUD SMITHERS
WILLIAM H. STEWART, SR
CHARLIE TATUM
SECRIST TEAGUE
BOON VAWTER
STEVE WHEAT
JOSEPH WATERMAN
EDGAR WATSON
JOE S. WEST
CHARLEY WHITE

The 40 causalities of the April 1918 fire at Central State Hospital were burned beyond recognition; only one boy was identified, and his family claimed his body for burial in a family cemetery. In 2015, it was difficult to find the unmarked grave, which turned out to measure 13 by 16 feet. This marker, dedicated in 2015, stands alone in the older part of the cemetery with no other markers in its vicinity. (CCHS.)

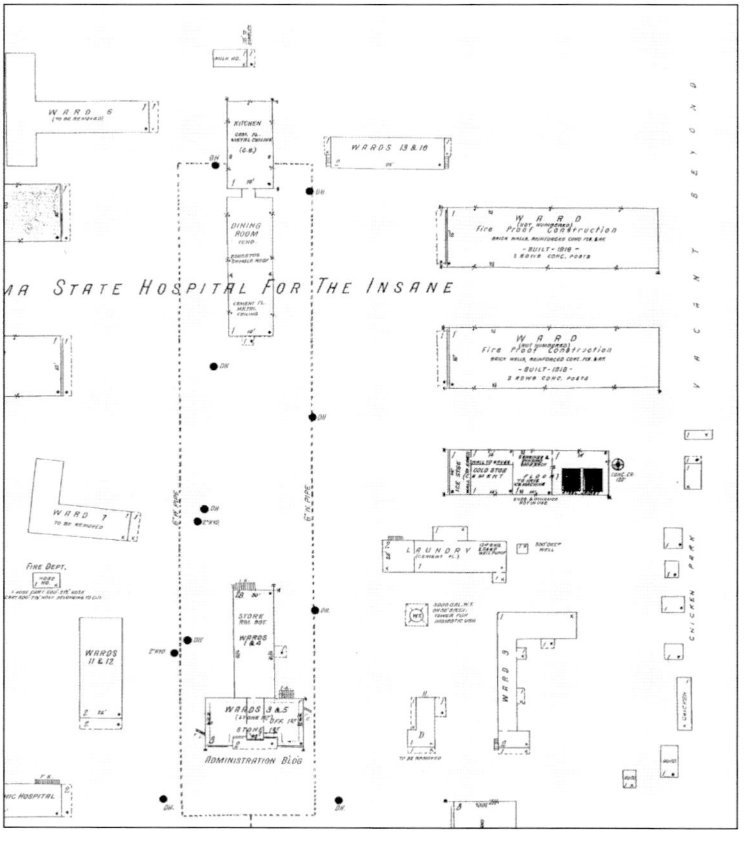

Within four months of the April 1918 fire, Central State Hospital had replaced wards 13, 14, and 15 and the dining hall, shown on this 1918 Sanborn insurance map, all of which were destroyed or damaged by the fire. The new building that housed wards 14 and 15 was a three-story structure made of brick, stone, and concrete; all of the new buildings were considered to be fireproof. The Oklahoma legislature appropriated $168,000 for this new construction. (CCHS.)

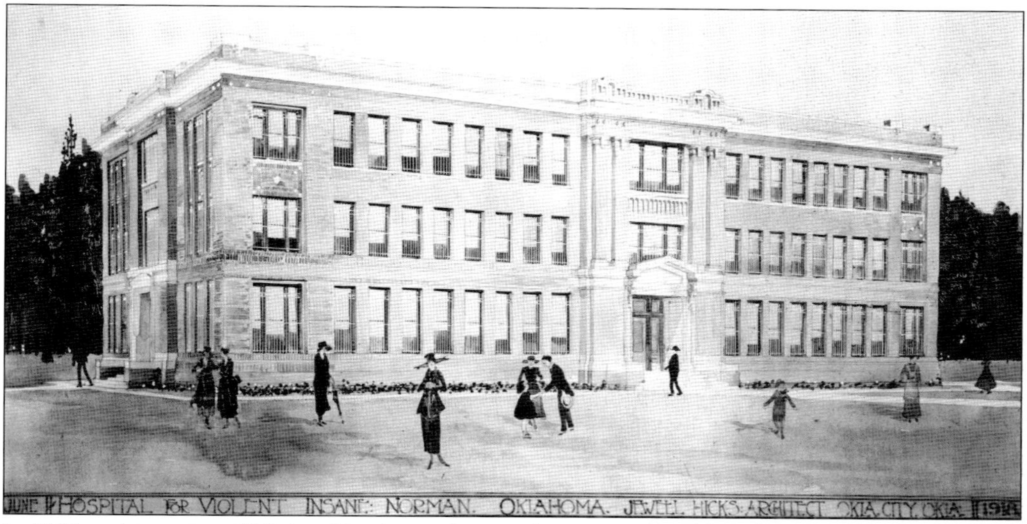
HOSPITAL FOR VIOLENT INSANE: NORMAN. OKLAHOMA. JEWELL HICKS: ARCHITECT OKLA. CITY, OKLA.

In 1918, architect Jewell Hicks offered a rendering of a new ward building for Central State Hospital; this building is most likely the one that housed wards 14 and 15. Many people considered Hicks to be Oklahoma's state architect because he designed many of the state's buildings, including the Oklahoma State Capitol and several structures at Oklahoma institutions and the University of Oklahoma. (OHS.)

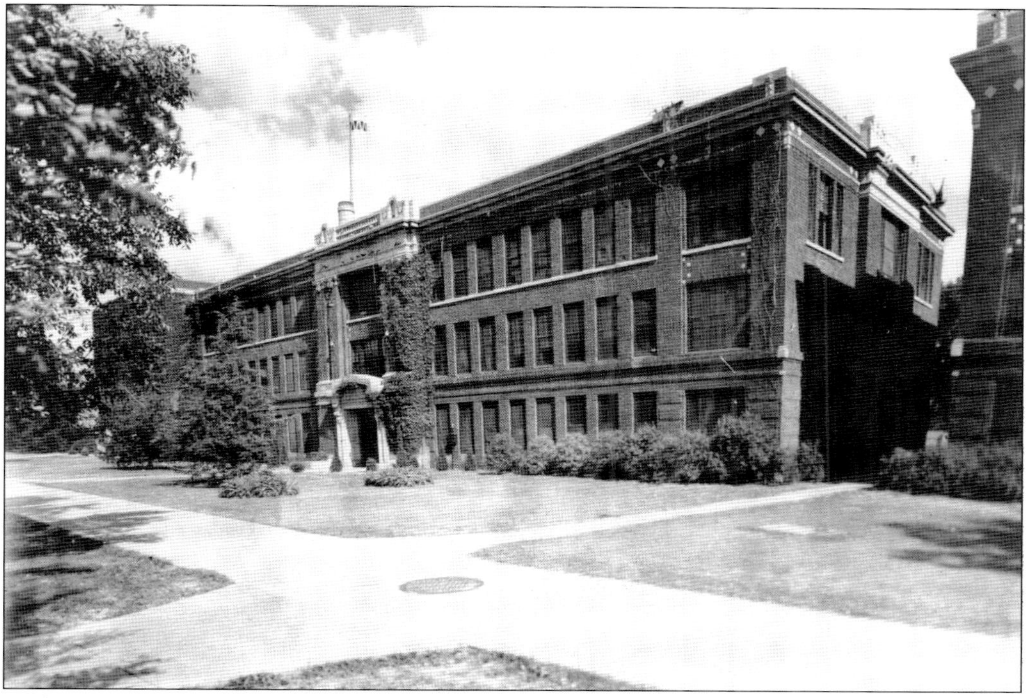

In the early 20th century, most buildings at Central State Hospital kept patients with different levels of mental illness in the same ward, meaning that those who were considered "violently insane" were housed with those who had milder mental disorders. This building, which followed Jewell Hicks's architectural drawing, is representative of the wards where patients lived in close proximity to one another. (CCHS.)

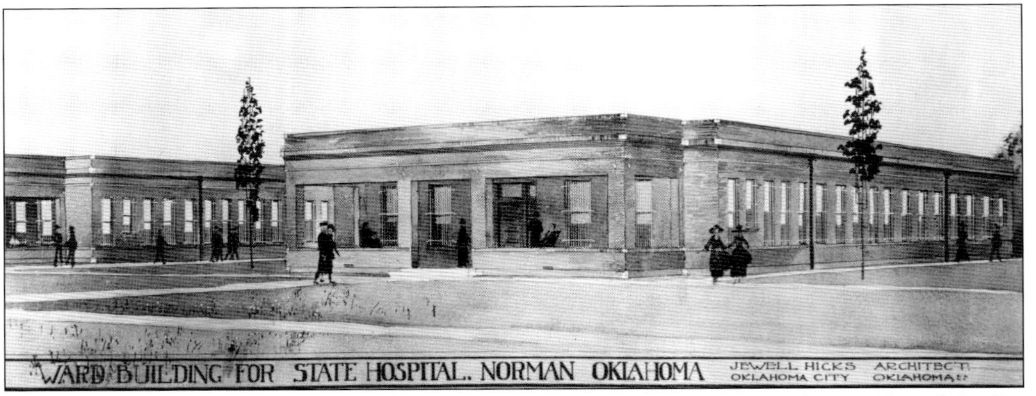

Architect Jewell Hicks also designed cottage-type ward buildings. Superintendent Dr. David Griffin believed that a more modern approach to treatment of mental disorders could be accomplished in a less threatening environment. This later design by Hicks represented Griffin's ideal that housing and treatment should correspond to a patient's illness, and that patients with similar mental disorders should be housed in the same area. (OHS.)

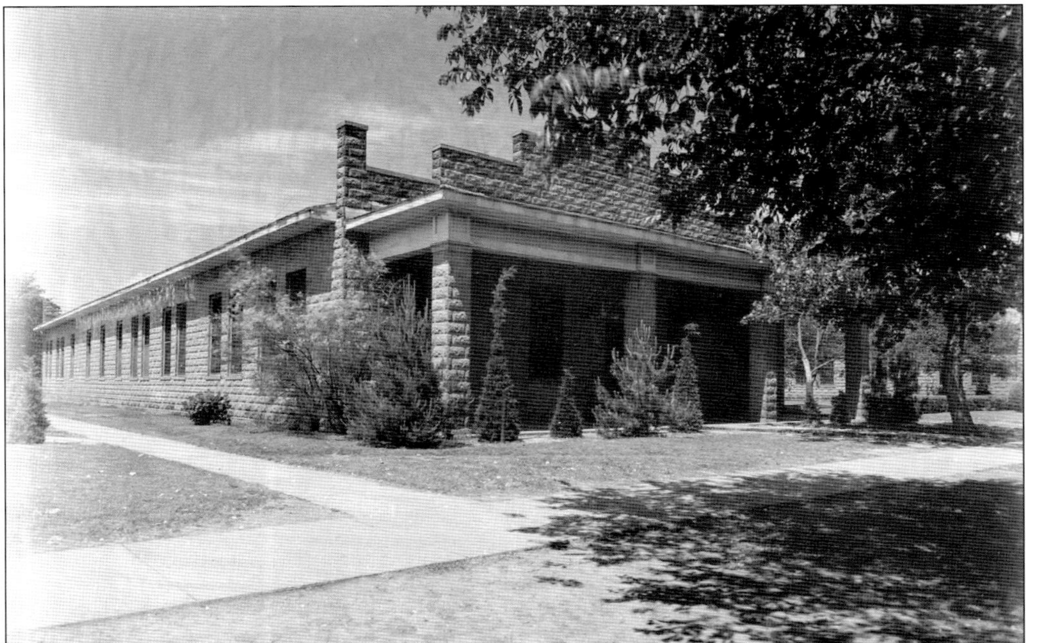

Jewell Hicks designed several cottages at Central State Hospital that Dr. Griffin believed were ideal for smaller groups of patients. The cottage design helped to create a campus-type atmosphere along with manicured lawns, mature trees, and flower gardens. The grounds included the administration building up front and cottages and other buildings bordering it. (CCHS.)

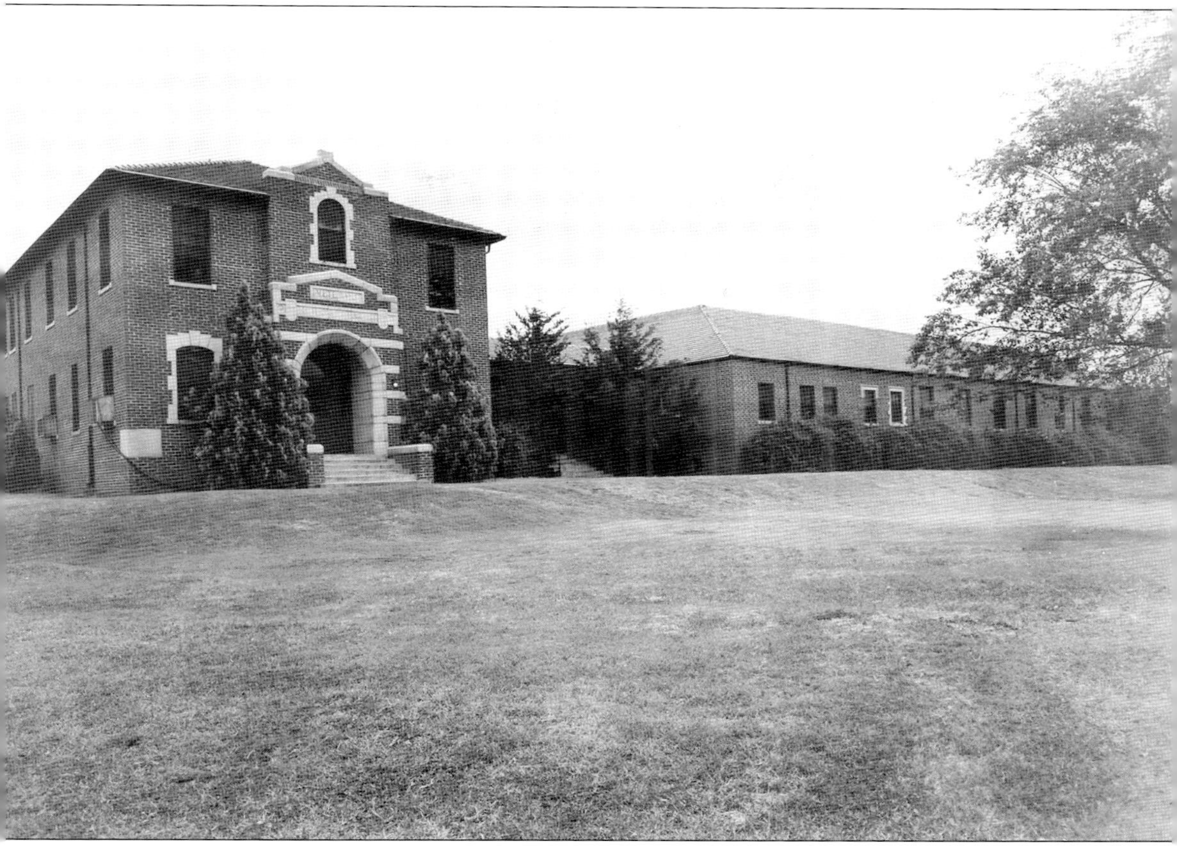

In 1920, over 20,000 veterans came home from the First World War sick and disabled. These men were housed in mental facilities and hospitals across the country. Over 200,000 American veterans campaigned for better facilities for the sick and injured. The American Legion supported a movement to find the veterans who came home from the war with mental trauma and were assigned to mental hospitals outside of their home regions. The federal government knew of 1,200 facilities that housed veterans after World War I. The American Legion made it a first priority to take a census and find the names and home states of the veterans housed in these hospitals. In 1922, there were 384 former servicemen from Oklahoma housed in 29 different hospitals scattered throughout 18 states. This image features one of the early veterans' buildings at Central State Hospital. (CCHS.)

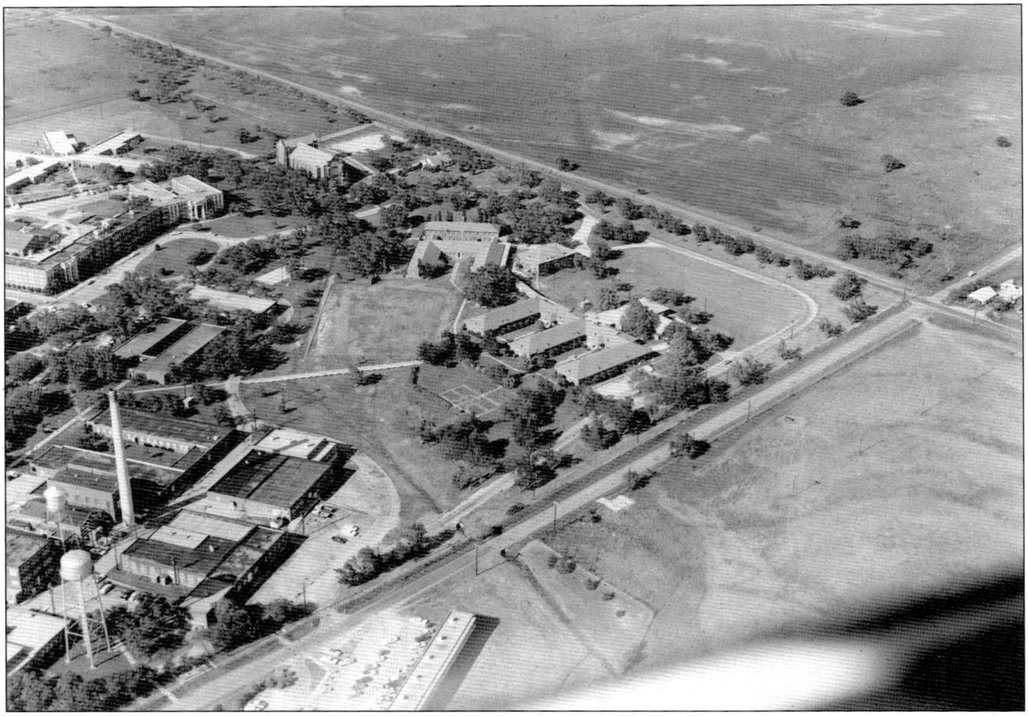

At Central State Hospital, the veterans' wards were at the northeast corner of the property, near the current intersection of Southeast Twelfth Avenue and Main Street. The Oklahoma legislature appropriated $2 million for the American Legion to build veterans' wards for servicemen who experienced physical and mental illnesses after World War I. In 1924, the veterans' ward was dedicated in a ceremony with the American Legion, the Legion Auxiliary, and the Soldiers Relief Commission. (OHS.)

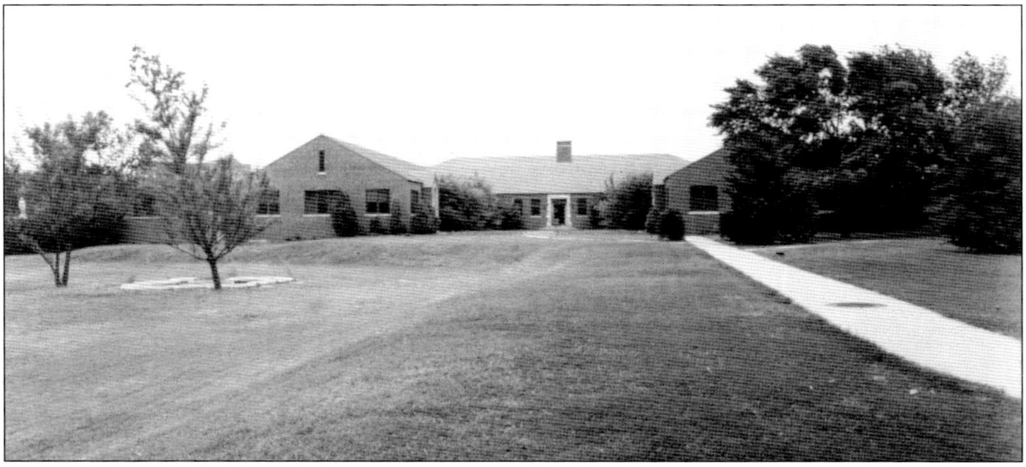

Superintendent Griffin outlined the need for the rehabilitation of veterans who were mentally ill, and he appreciated the new buildings the state constructed at Central State Hospital. Griffin also emphasized that a new building was not enough; to properly rehabilitate these veterans, the state needed to appropriate enough funds for professional staff members who could help the men recover. (CCHS.)

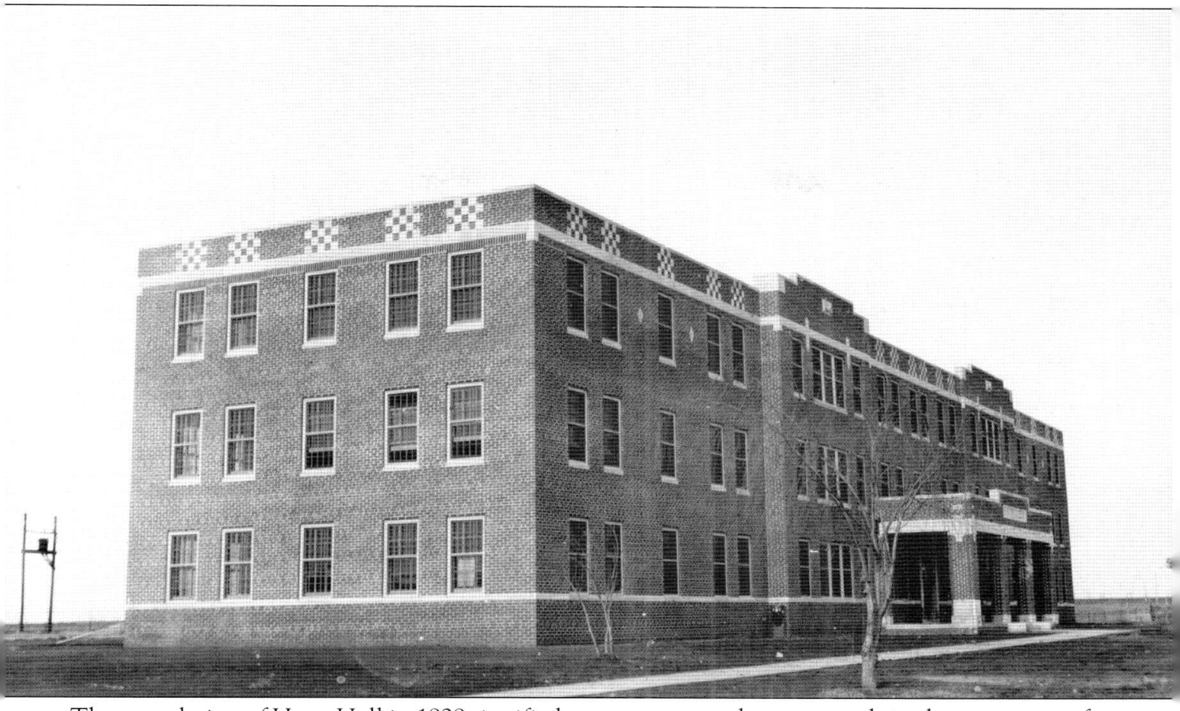

The completion of Hope Hall in 1929 signified a new, more modern approach in the treatment of mental illness at Central State. Dr. Griffin believed that most patients with mental illness could be cured with modern techniques. The new psychiatric building gave each patient renewed hope, according to Griffin. Each new patient was evaluated at Hope Hall, and a course of treatment was prescribed, such as hydrotherapy or electrotherapy. Those who could not be treated were assigned an appropriate ward for their stage of illness. Griffin noted that "they were cared for as tenderly as possible, without hope of permanent relief from their afflictions." When Hope Hall was completed, it had a 150-bed capacity, along with 30 nurses and six doctors. Griffin expected to spend another $50,000 on the latest equipment used in psychiatric care. The completion of Hope Hall brought some resolution to a 29-year effort by Griffin to provide outstanding psychiatric care in Oklahoma. When Hope Hall was completed, it was one of the best treatment facilities in the country. (OHS.)

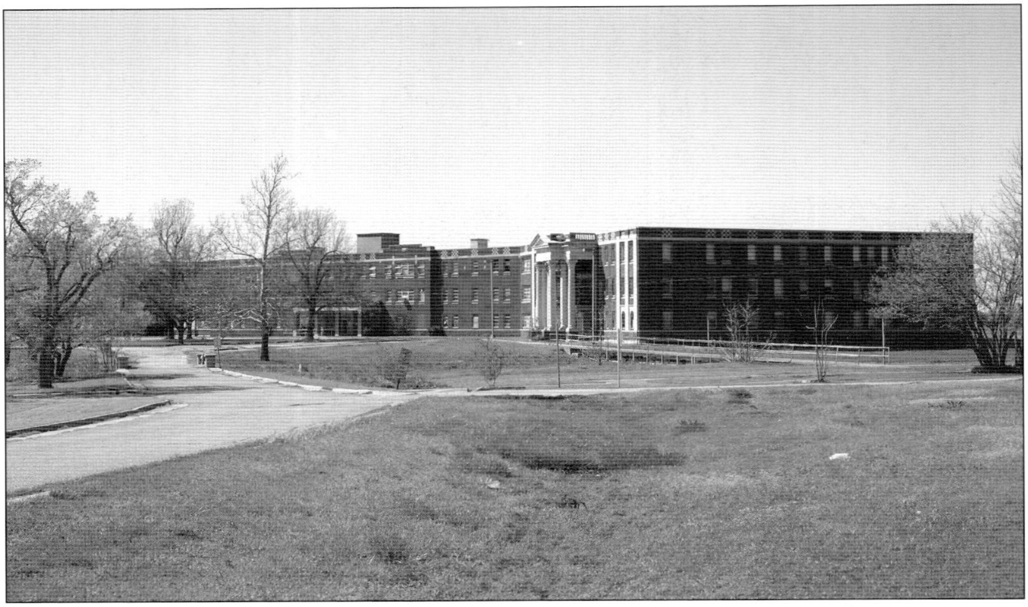

In 1930, Central State Hospital was still 30 percent overcrowded. Even after the acquisition of state funds for 100 new beds, superintendent Griffin still had to house patients in hallways. The state lunacy board asked the county judge to admit only the violently insane. Temporary relief came with a $150,000 appropriation for a new ward, which was added on to Hope Hall. The east side of Hope Hall (at left) was completed in 1931. (CCHS.)

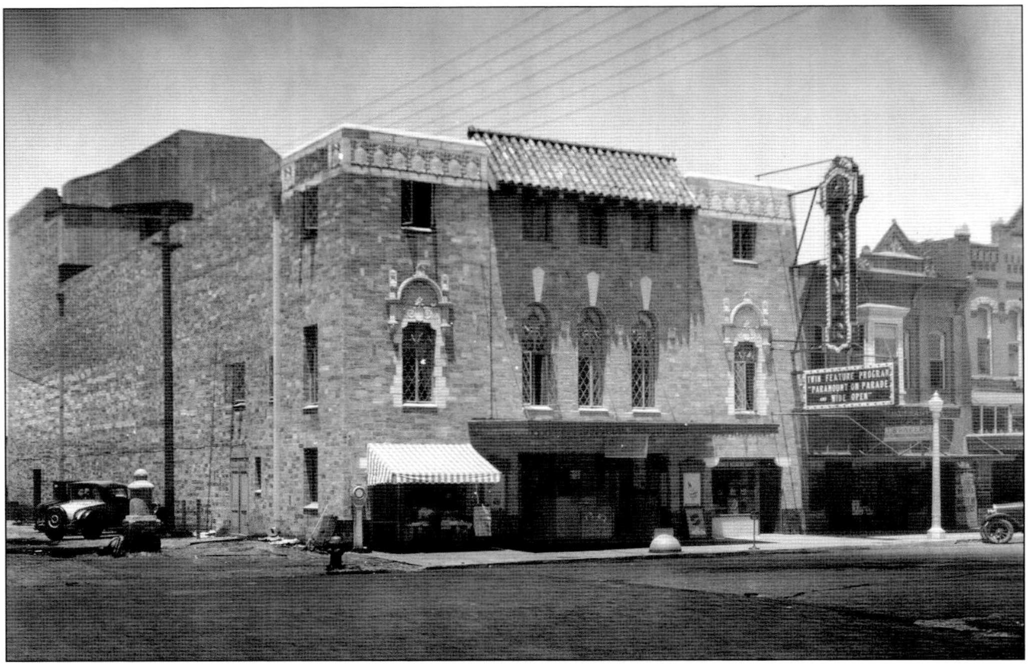

The Sooner Theater on Main Street in downtown Norman was built in 1929, the same time Hope Hall was finished at Central State Hospital. Both buildings represented the prosperity and growth of the town and its main institution. (CCHS.)

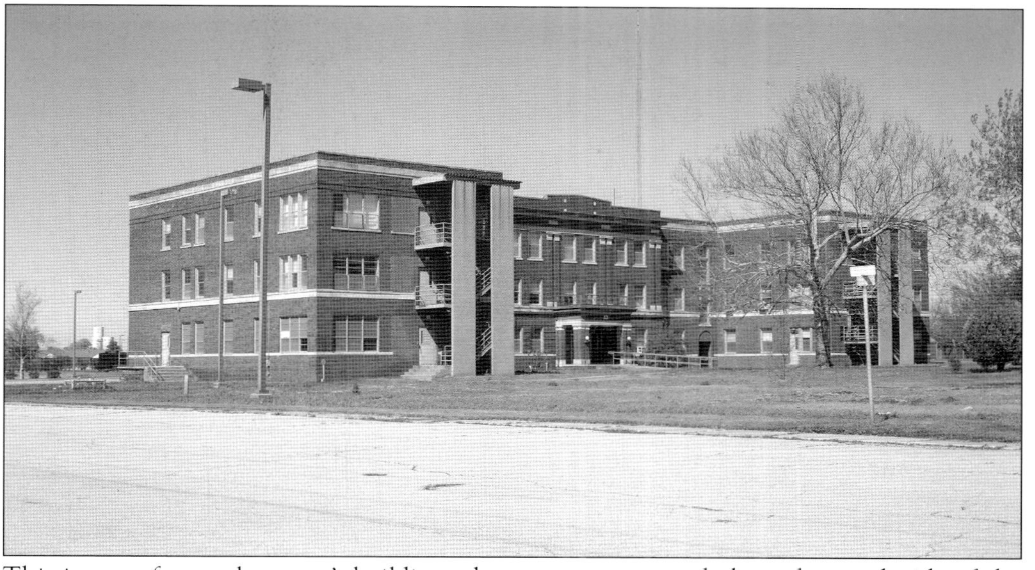

This is one of several women's buildings that were constructed along the north side of the administration building in the 1930s. Doctors determined that there was a significant difference between mental illness in men and women. At that time, physicians considered women to be more out of control in expressing their emotions; they tended to be hysterical and needed more restraint than men. The women's wards were also more crowded. (CCHS.)

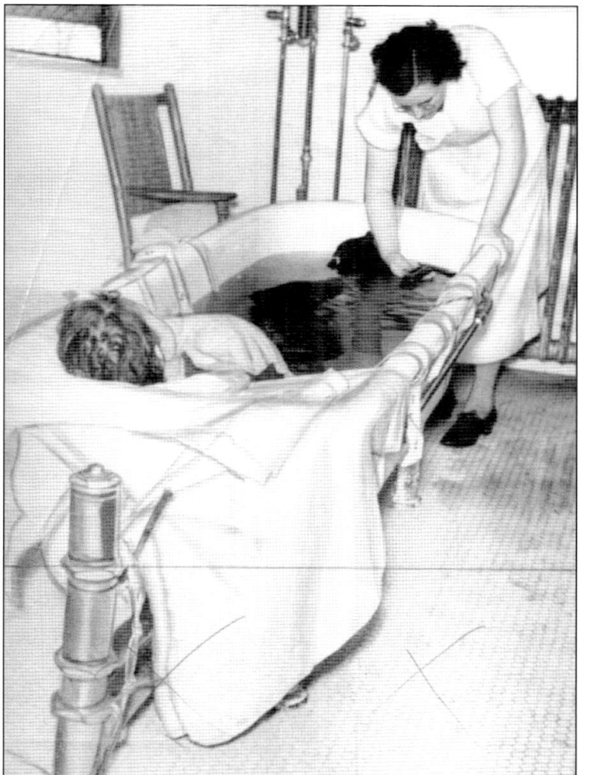

The continue flow bath was used for delirious or exceptionally excitable women. To quiet patients, an attendant laid them down in a canvas hammock in the bath, where they were submerged to the ears. There was a continual flow of 97-degree water. A patient stayed in the bath all day, and some stayed in for two or three days. Men had a bath in their ward as well. (OHS.)

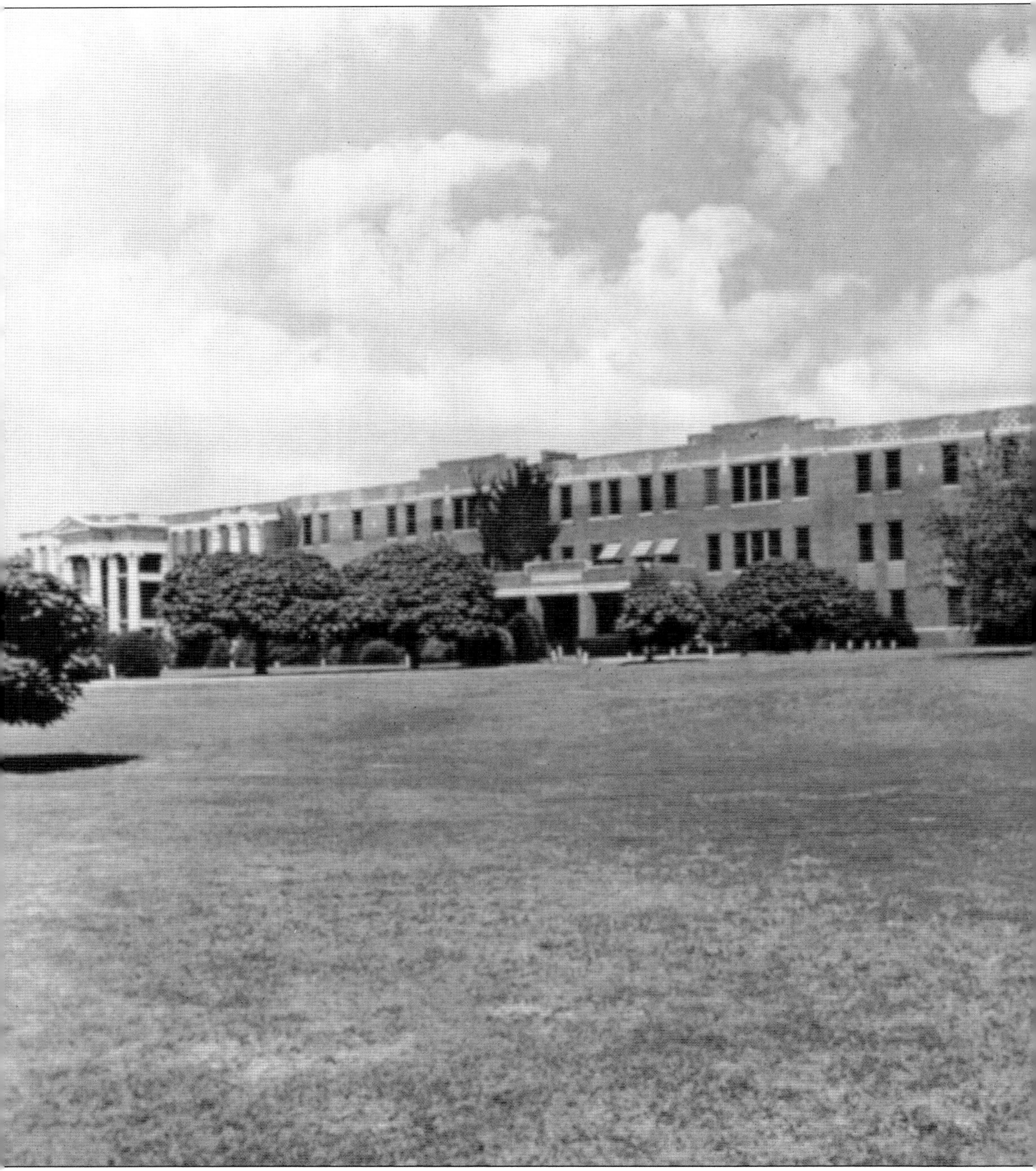

In 1936, the State of Oklahoma appropriated funds to complete Hope Hall, which is pictured here. The original middle section continued to be the center for the admission and evaluation of new patients. Along with the continue flow bath, another new treatment included insulin shock therapy. Doctors used insulin shock therapy with the thought that insulin would shock the patient back to sanity. Another controversial treatment was sterilization. In keeping with the eugenics movement of the early 20th century, Oklahoma passed legislation in 1931 and again in

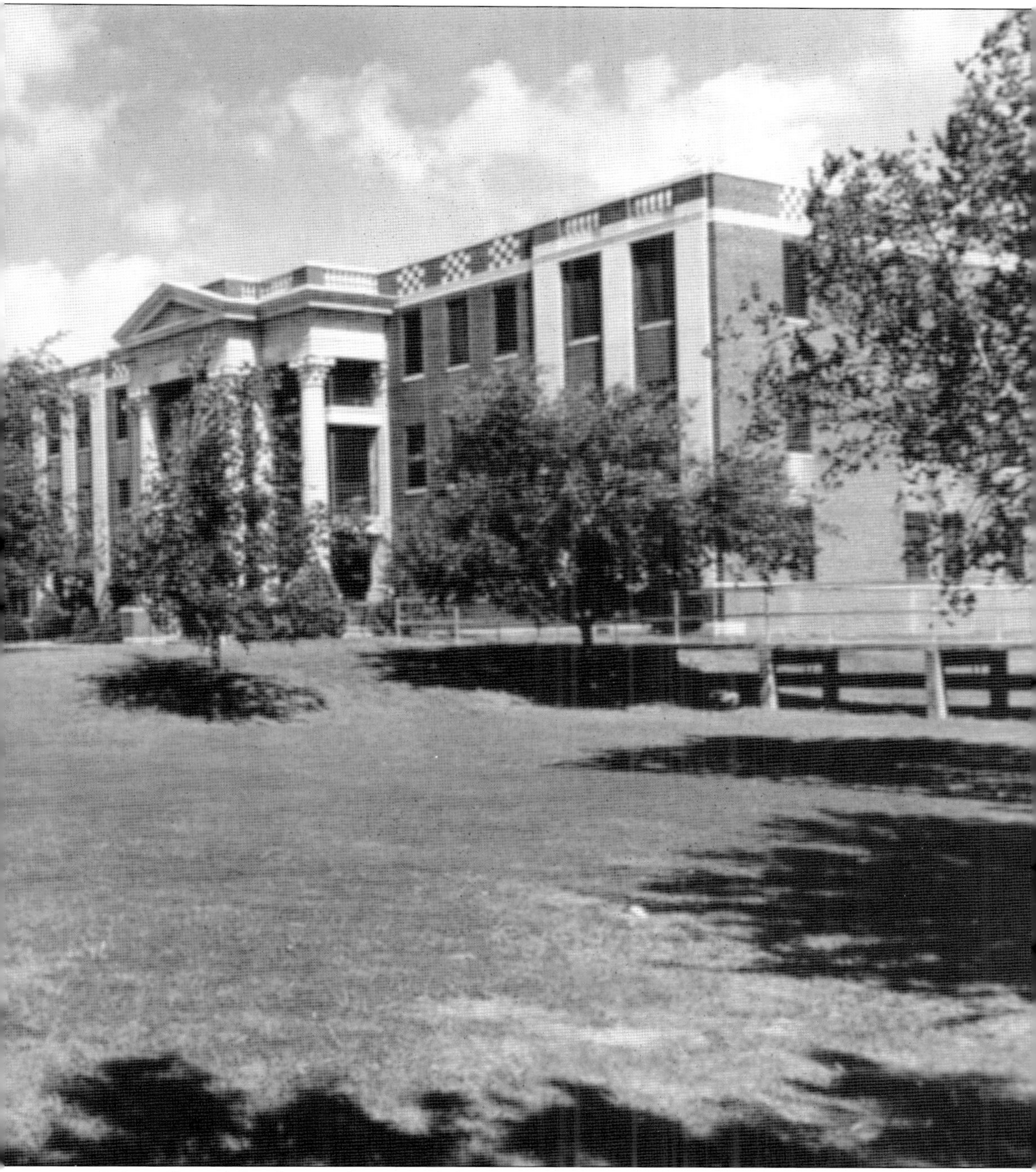

1935 that allowed for the sterilization of the mentally ill and of criminals in the state's prisons. Central State superintendent Griffin needed court approval for the sterilization of patients, and the court generally approved his recommendations. In all treatments, the general idea was to move the patient from insanity to sanity and eventually back home to their families. The second floor in the east wing was for female patients, and the second floor of the west wing housed male patients. Most therapy treatments were on the third floor. (CCHS.)

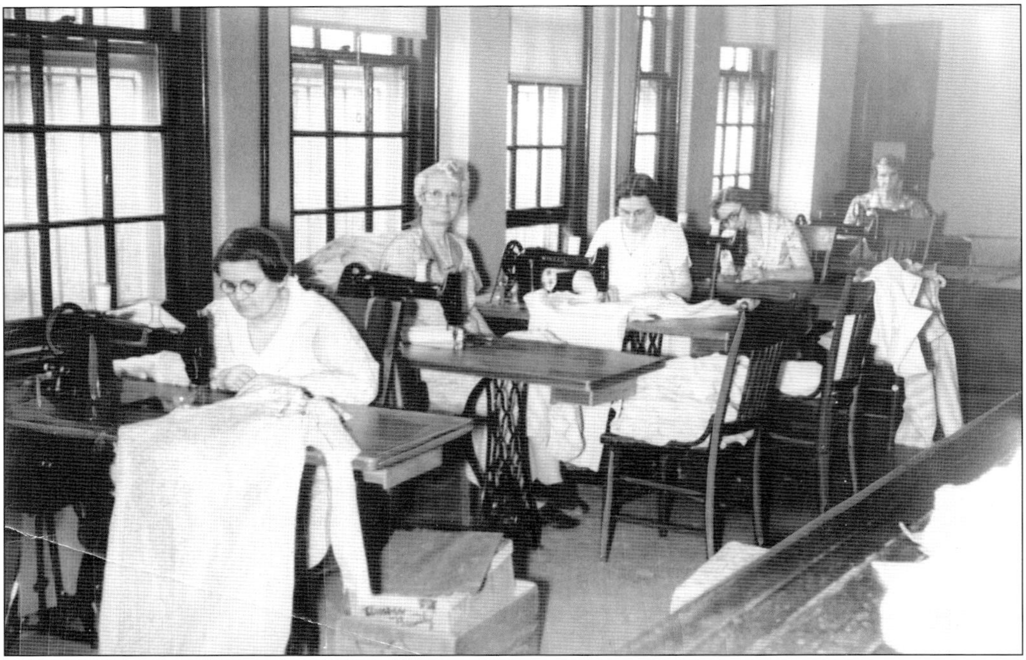

Dr. Griffin considered that most of the patients at Central State Hospital, through various treatments, could be cured of their disorders and moved back into society. One step in returning patients to their homes was some kind of vocational and household training. The women pictured here in 1936 were taught how to use a sewing machine to produce necessary items for the hospital. (OHS.)

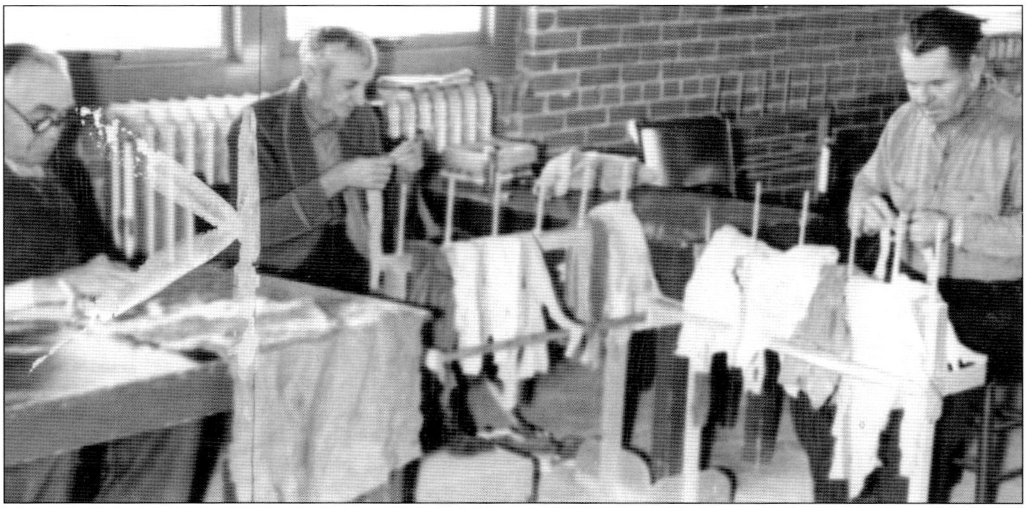

Male patients at Central State were also given the opportunity to be creative. They worked in the hospital industry building, where they used discarded items such as prune boxes, potato sacks, and even silk stockings donated by women's clubs to create objects of art. Outside observers noted the interest and enjoyment the men held for their crafts. These men are preparing materials for a loom. (OHS.)

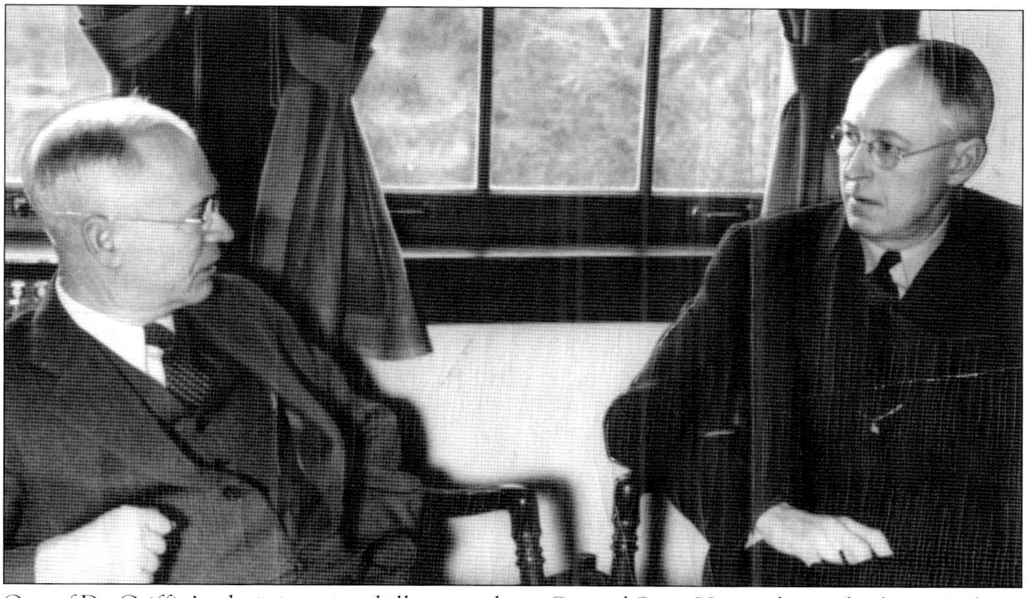

One of Dr. Griffin's administrative skills was to keep Central State Hospital out of politics. Perhaps his ability to do so contributed to his longevity as superintendent of the hospital. In 1935, Griffin (left), who was then the hospital's superintendent, had been on staff for 37 years. Dr. J.J. Gable (right), assistant superintendent, was at the Norman institution for 22 years. (OHS.)

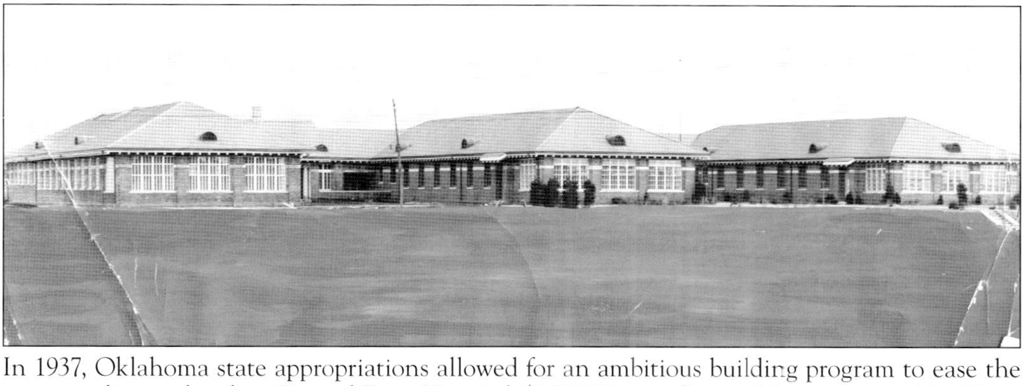

In 1937, Oklahoma state appropriations allowed for an ambitious building program to ease the overcrowding and update Central State Hospital: $269,000 was allocated for a new ward building, and the same amount was approved for another ward in 1938. The appropriations also included $100,000 to restore the dining hall and kitchen and $175,000 for the power plant. These buildings were the most modern yet at the hospital. (OHS.)

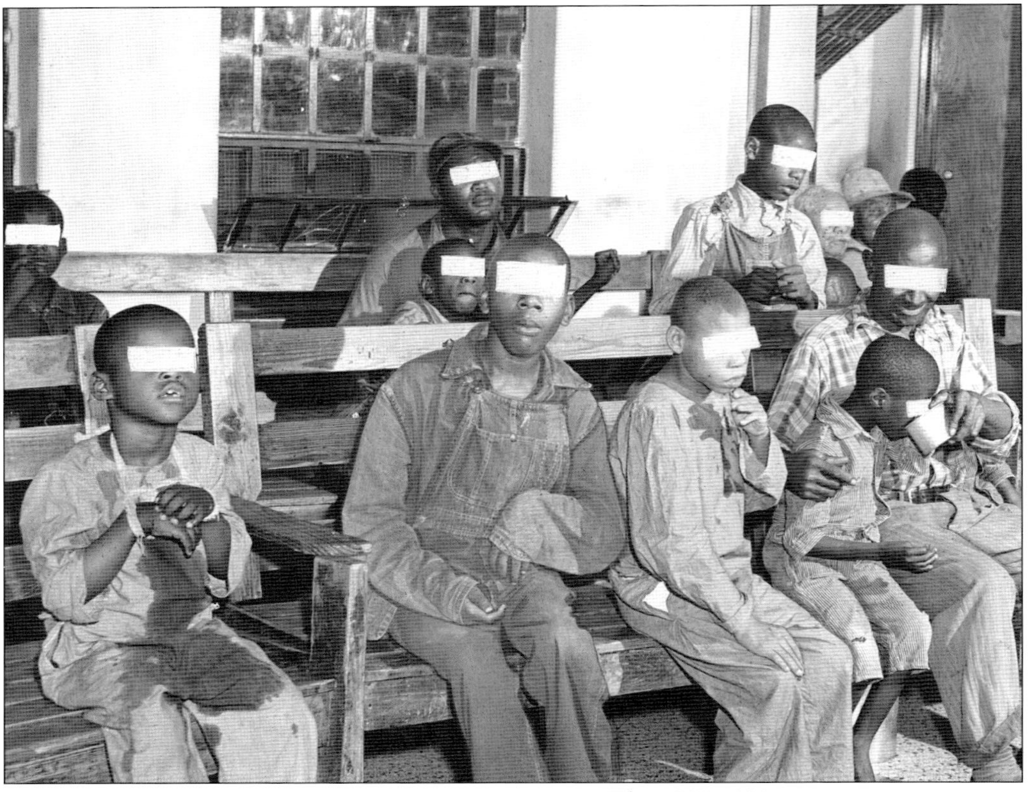

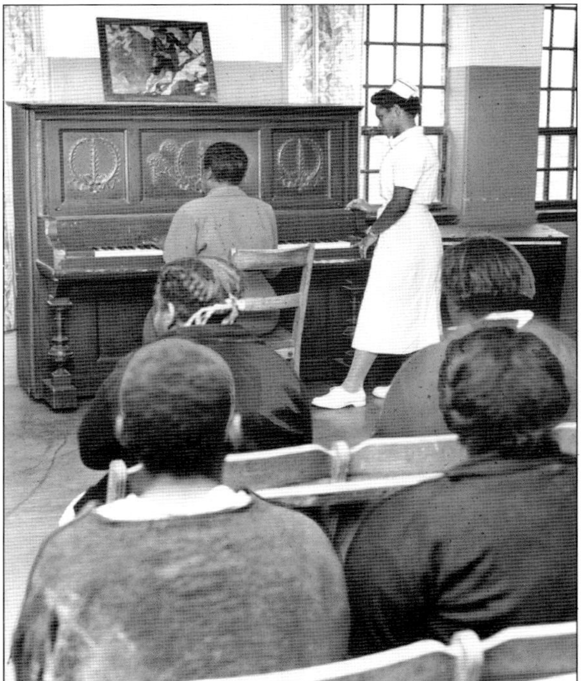

The 1937–1938 construction at Central State Hospital provided more room for incoming patients. The relocation of Black patients to the newly constructed Taft State Hospital for the Negro Insane also opened up more room at the Norman asylum. The caption for this image from the *Daily Oklahoman* reads, "A dreary dayroom scene in the State Hospital for the Negro Insane at Taft." (OHS.)

Taft State Hospital for the Negro Insane was eight miles west of Muskogee, Oklahoma. Taft was built by the state in 1934 and was operated by Black doctors, nurses, and other staff. The caption for this image from the *Daily Oklahoman* reads, "The patient at the piano is a talented musician." The same programs instituted at other mental institutions in the state were instituted at Taft. (OHS.)

One of the measures that Central State Hospital superintendent Dr. Griffin believed would facilitate mental well-being for patients was a place on hospital grounds that offered recreational and spiritual guidance. The economic depression of the 1930s offered Griffin the opportunity to obtain the financial resources and the labor he needed to realize his goal. This is a front view of the construction of the American Legion Memorial Chapel in 1936. (OHS.)

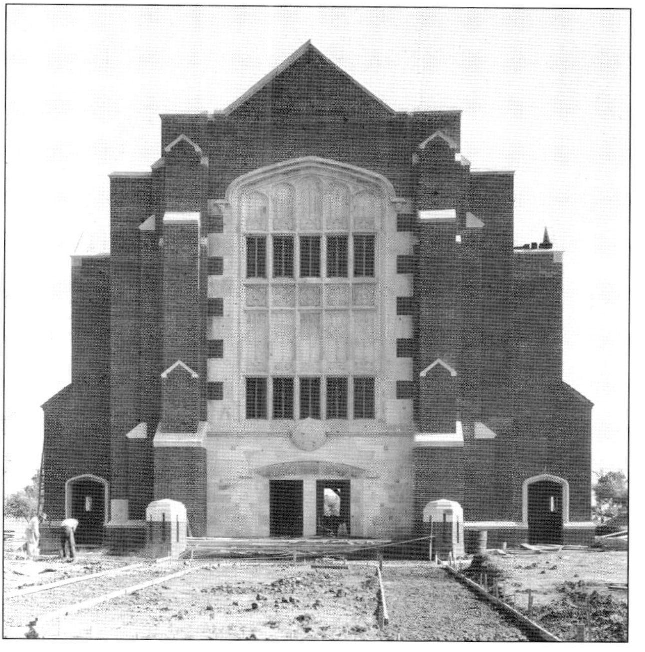

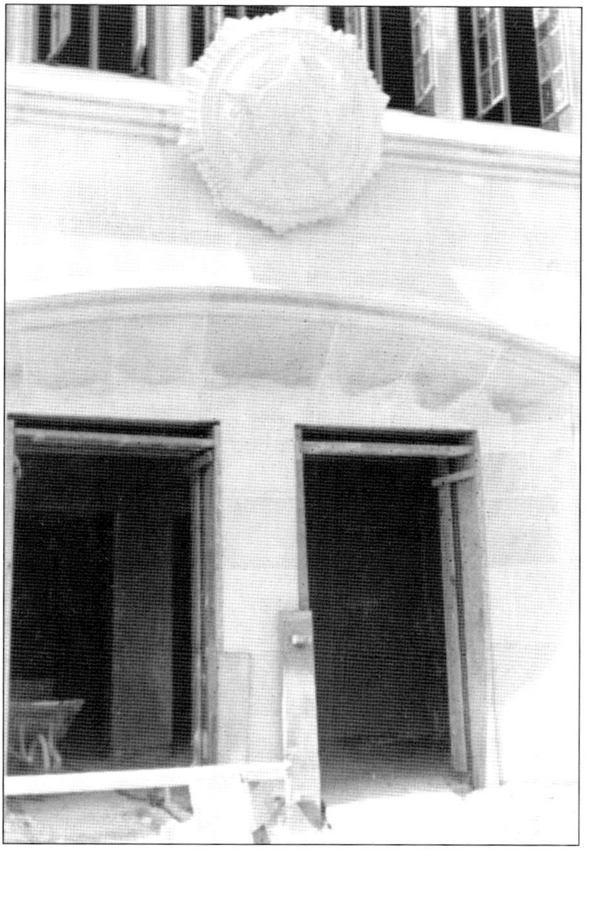

The original funding for the American Legion Memorial Chapel was a 1929 state appropriation of $1,308,500 to Central State Hospital that included $85,000 for the chapel. However, it was not until 1936 that work began on the chapel; that year was when Pres. Franklin D. Roosevelt's New Deal program, the Public Works Administration, offered matching funds for projects in Oklahoma. (OHS.)

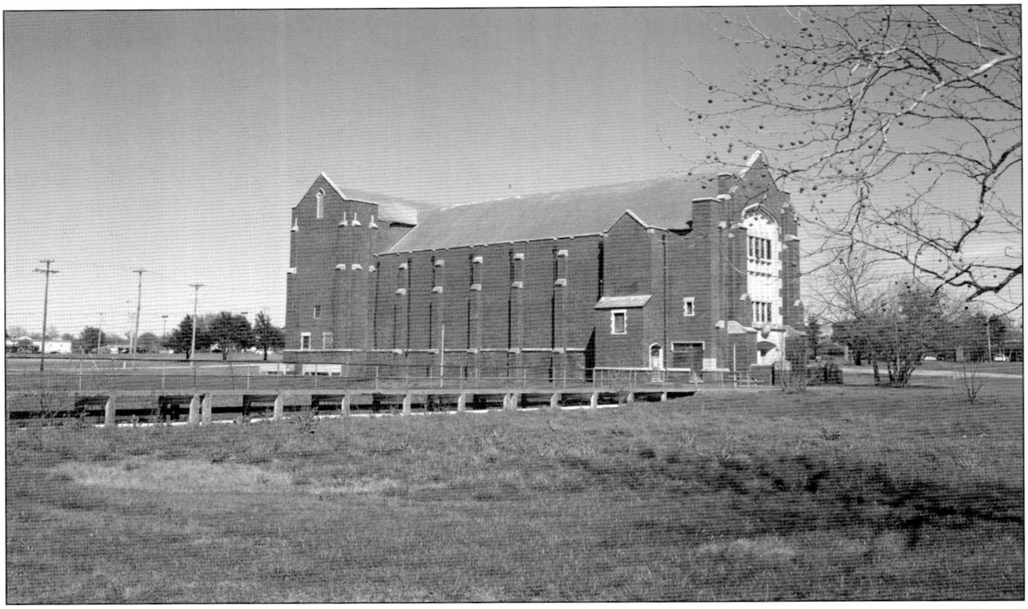

Public Works Administration programs provided a financial stimulus and jobs to states and local communities. Government money was a matching grant, which meant that states and communities provided a share of the project financing. The Fletcher O'Dell Pledger American Legion Post also donated $16,000 toward the construction of the chapel at Central State Hospital, and the chapel became known as the American Legion Memorial Chapel. (CCHS.)

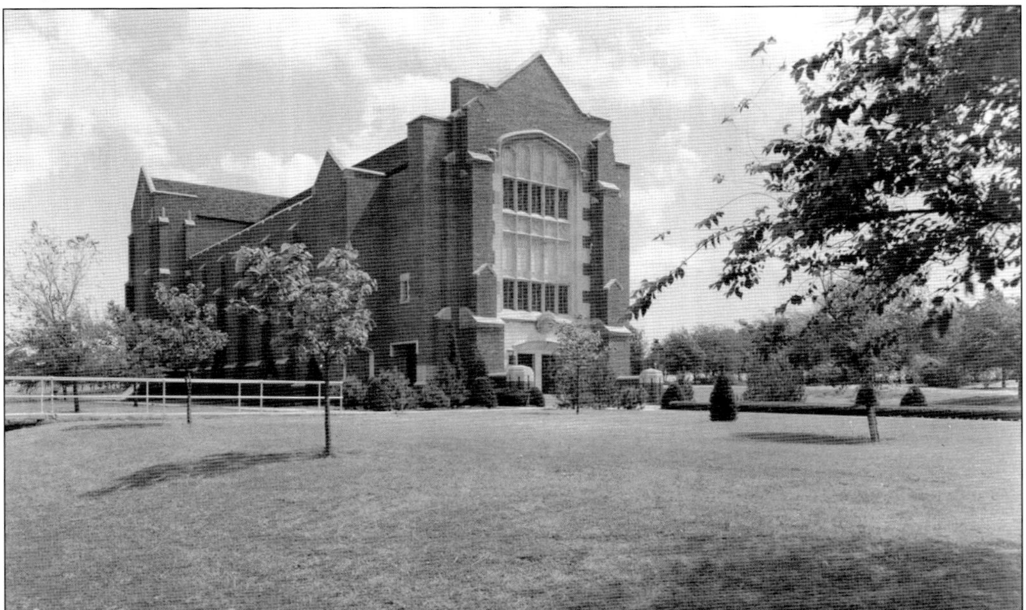

The chapel included a large auditorium that held 1,500 people. The chapel was used for church services and recreation; the facility had a stage, screen, and projector. The building encompassed what Dr. Griffin had envisioned in 1929. In 2020, the chapel stands as one of the few structures that remain out of the 29 buildings that were constructed in the early 20th century. (CCHS.)

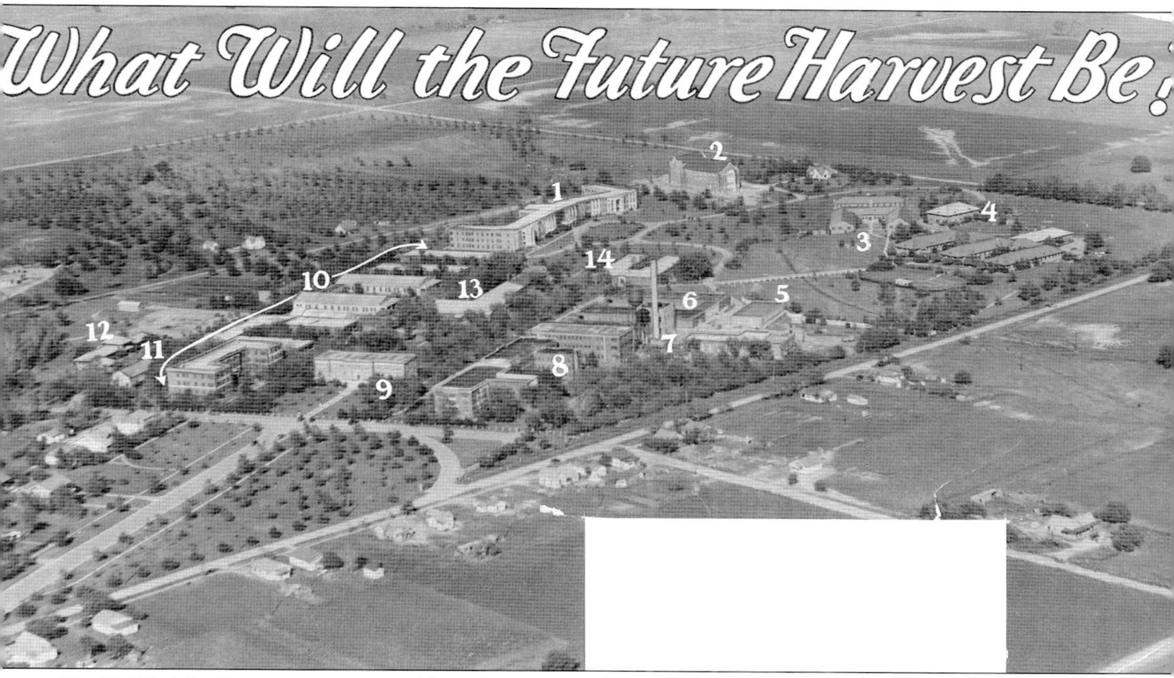

Dr. Griffin's building program could not keep up with the number of patients admitted during the Great Depression. The hospital became a place where some migrants, lacking shelter and food, could find room and board. In 1936, there were 2,700 patients at Central State Hospital. The women's wards were the most overcrowded. An average of 112 patients entered the institution each month, while only 90 left. Eventually, some migrants received government checks and left the institution. This photograph accompanied an article in the *Daily Oklahoman* and shows the buildings that existed in the 1930s, including Hope Hall (1), the American Legion Memorial Chapel (2), the veterans' wards (3), the men's industrial building (4), a storeroom for food and supplies (5), the men's ward (6), the hospital laundry (7), the women's ward (8), the administration building (9), the women's industrial building (11), tuberculosis and pellagra wards (12), the main dining hall and kitchen (13), and the ward devoted to epileptic patients (14). (OHS.)

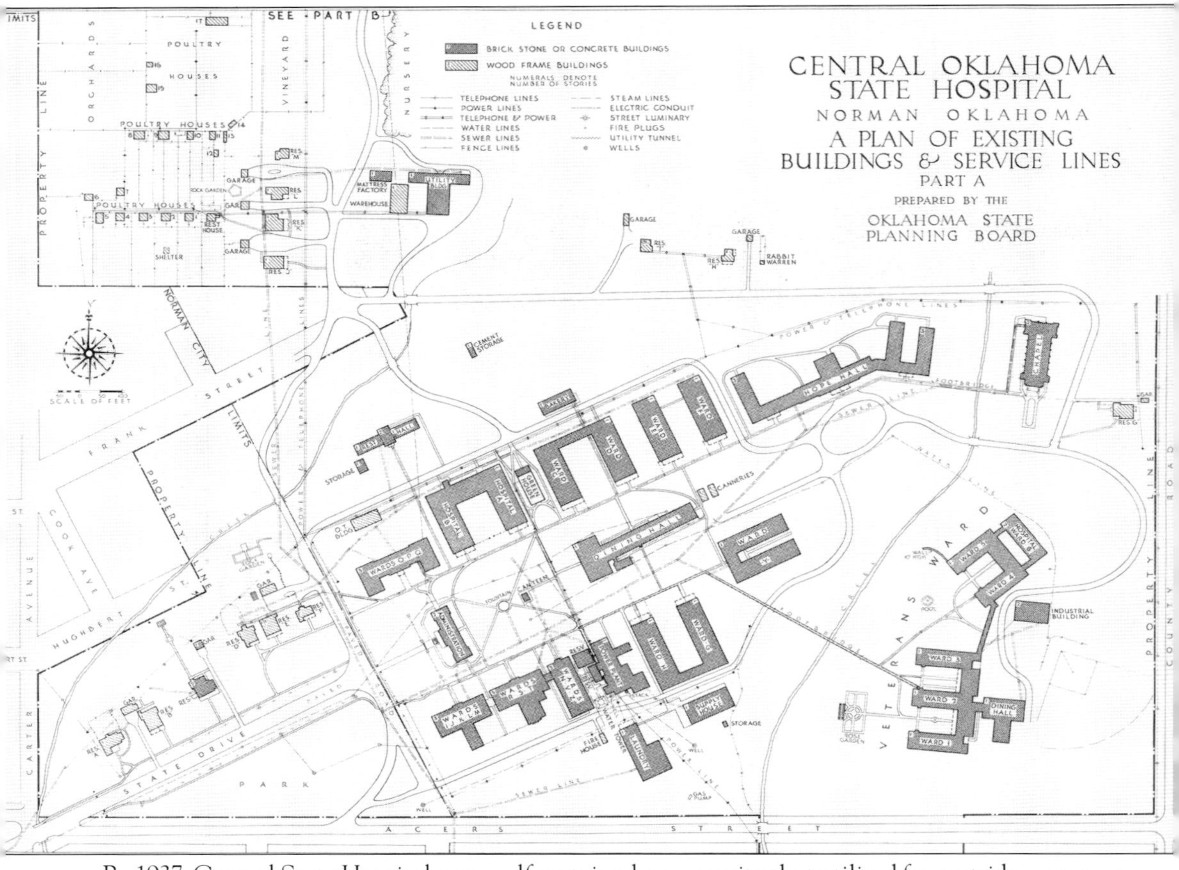

By 1937, Central State Hospital was a self-sustained community that utilized few outside resources except state funding that was needed for the construction of new buildings and the maintenance of existing buildings. The hospital owned three farms in Cleveland County that helped to make it self-sufficient. This map shows 26 buildings, including veterans' wards, storage and supply buildings, the fire department, a water and power facility, a greenhouse, a bakery, the industrial building, and a hospital. There were also six residences for doctors and staff. The map shows that Central State Hospital was just outside the boundaries of Norman. The residences for the superintendent and professional staff were on State Drive in the city. Most of Central State was in Cleveland County. The veterans' center and hospital are at the northeast corner of the hospital property. (OHS.)

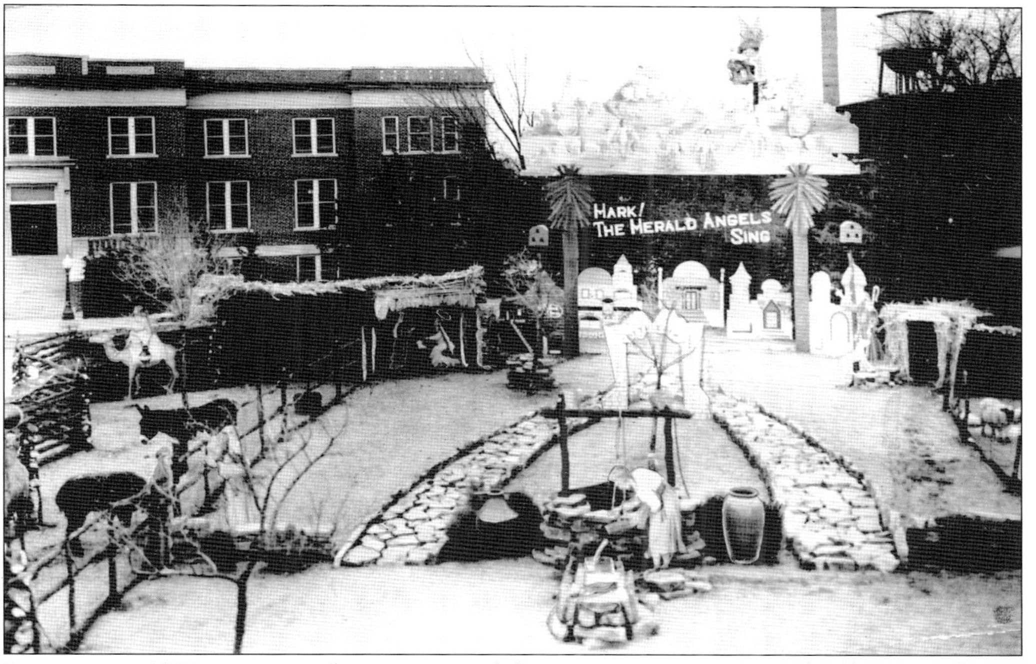

Beginning in 1937, patients in the occupational therapy program constructed a Christmas display that attracted visitors from around Oklahoma and also received national attention. One hundred patients started work on the display in June for its opening on December 20. In 1938, some 27,000 people saw the display. The 1939 display was called "Hark! The Herald Angels Sing," and the hospital expected 50,000 visitors that year. (OHS.)

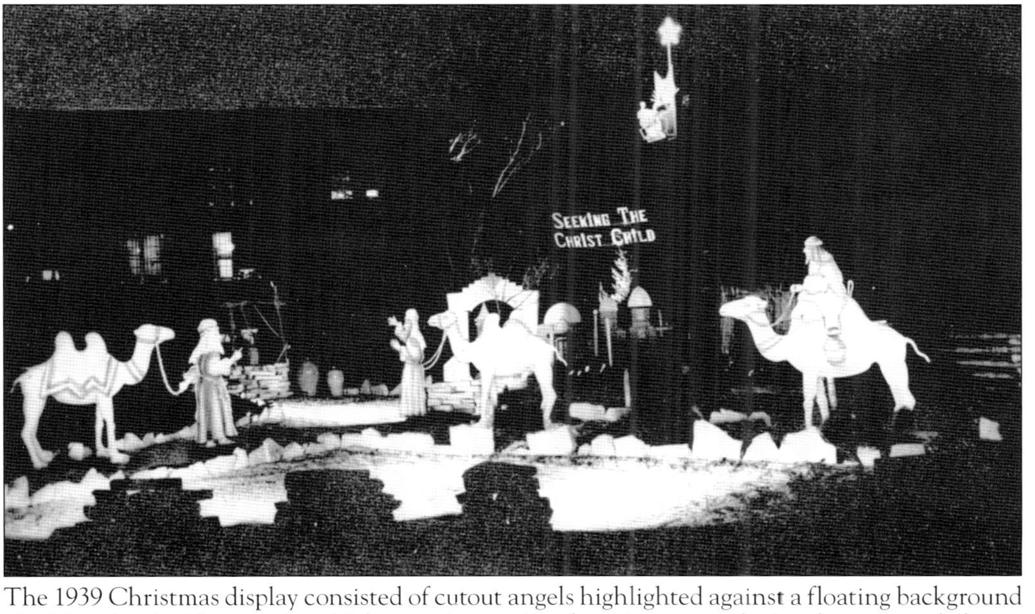

The 1939 Christmas display consisted of cutout angels highlighted against a floating background of white clouds. The angels, which were in continual motion, were depicted as suspended over Bethlehem. The patients added realism to the display with three camels borrowed from the Oklahoma City Zoo. Music was also made to emanate from the angels. (OHS.)

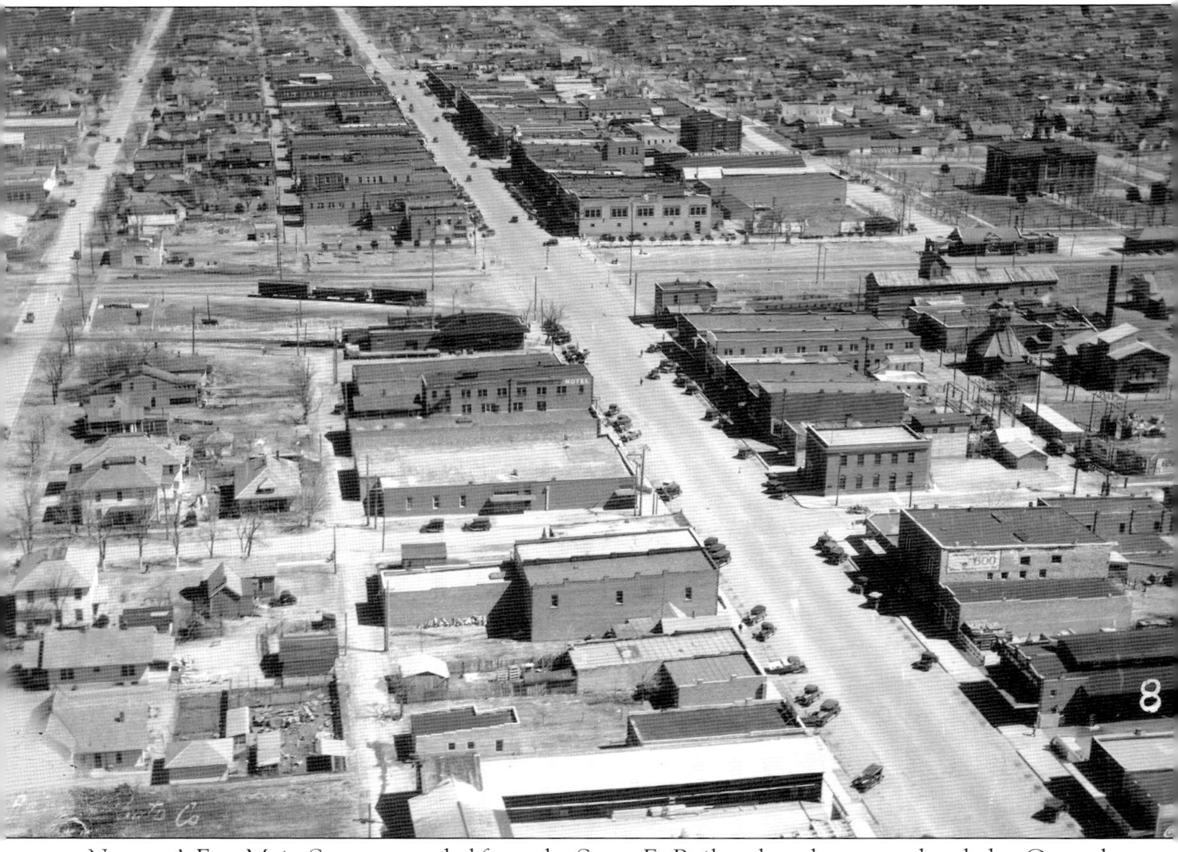

Norman's East Main Street extended from the Santa Fe Railroad tracks east and ended at Central State Hospital. Although the hospital was a major component of the economic success of the town, few of Norman's citizens knew what the conditions were inside the buildings, which were surrounded by parklike lawns and landscaping. However, by the 1940s, concerned citizens and politicians began taking a look inside. (CCHS.)

Three

Misery and Overcrowding 1940s

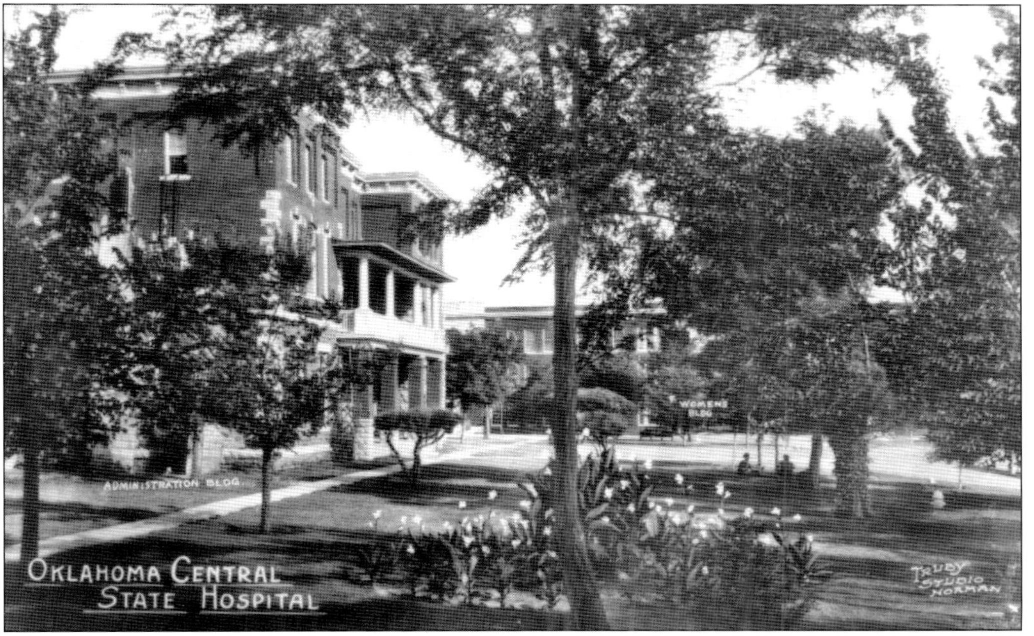

In the 1940s, psychiatric experts were concerned about worsening conditions in mental institutions in the United States. Mike Gorman, reporter for the *Daily Oklahoman*, investigated Central State Hospital in 1946. At first, the beautifully groomed grounds deceived Gorman. After a two-week investigation inside the hospital's buildings, he reported on the appalling conditions in which patients lived. Gorman called for public awareness and increased funding to ameliorate the problems. (OHS.)

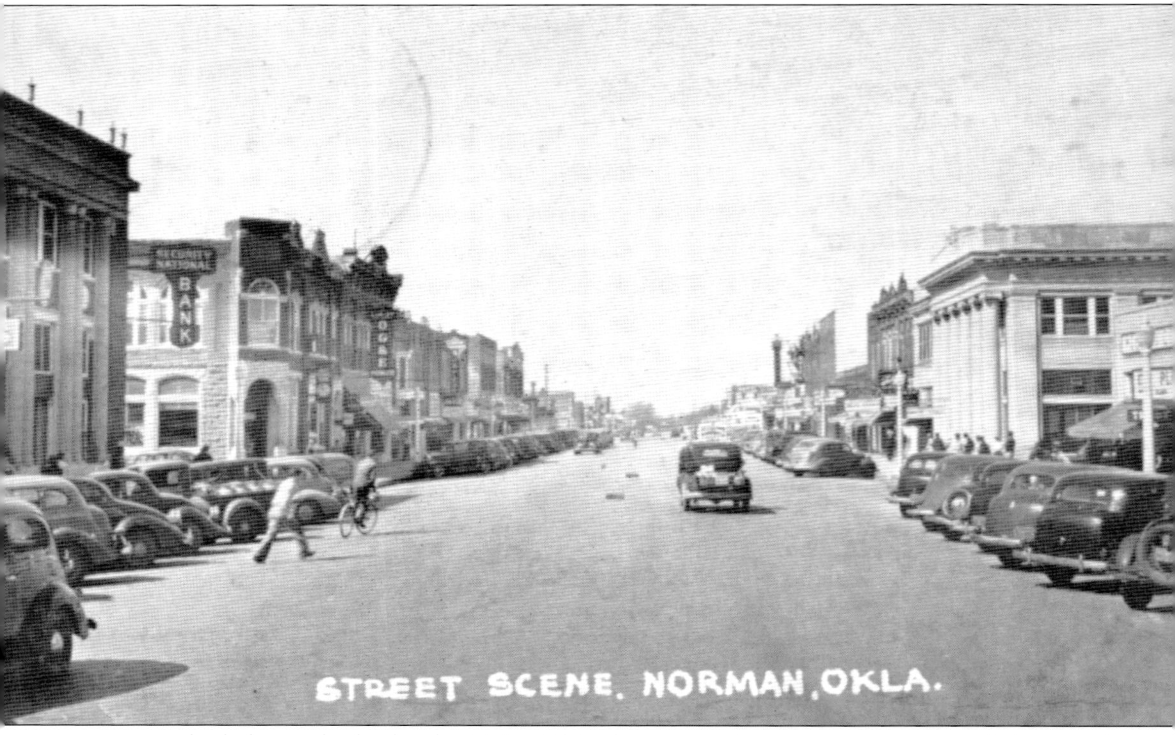

Norman had changed a lot by the 1940s. This change was largely due to the establishment of two naval facilities in the city. The Navy built a naval air station at the newly established Max Westheimer airfield north of town. South of town, adjacent to the University of Oklahoma, was the Naval Air Technical Training Center. The two bases brought 20,000 people to town for over six years. The benefits to Norman included updated infrastructure, including septic systems, water wells, and roads. Another benefit was the economic stimulus provided by the paychecks of servicemen and women who made purchases in the local economy. Norman had suffered in the Great Depression. By the 1940s, the influx of people with jobs and money had turned it into a prosperous and active town. When *Daily Oklahoman* reporter Michael Gorman entered the gates of Central State Hospital in 1946, at first, he saw this prosperity. But when he went into the asylum, he witnessed despair. (CCHS.)

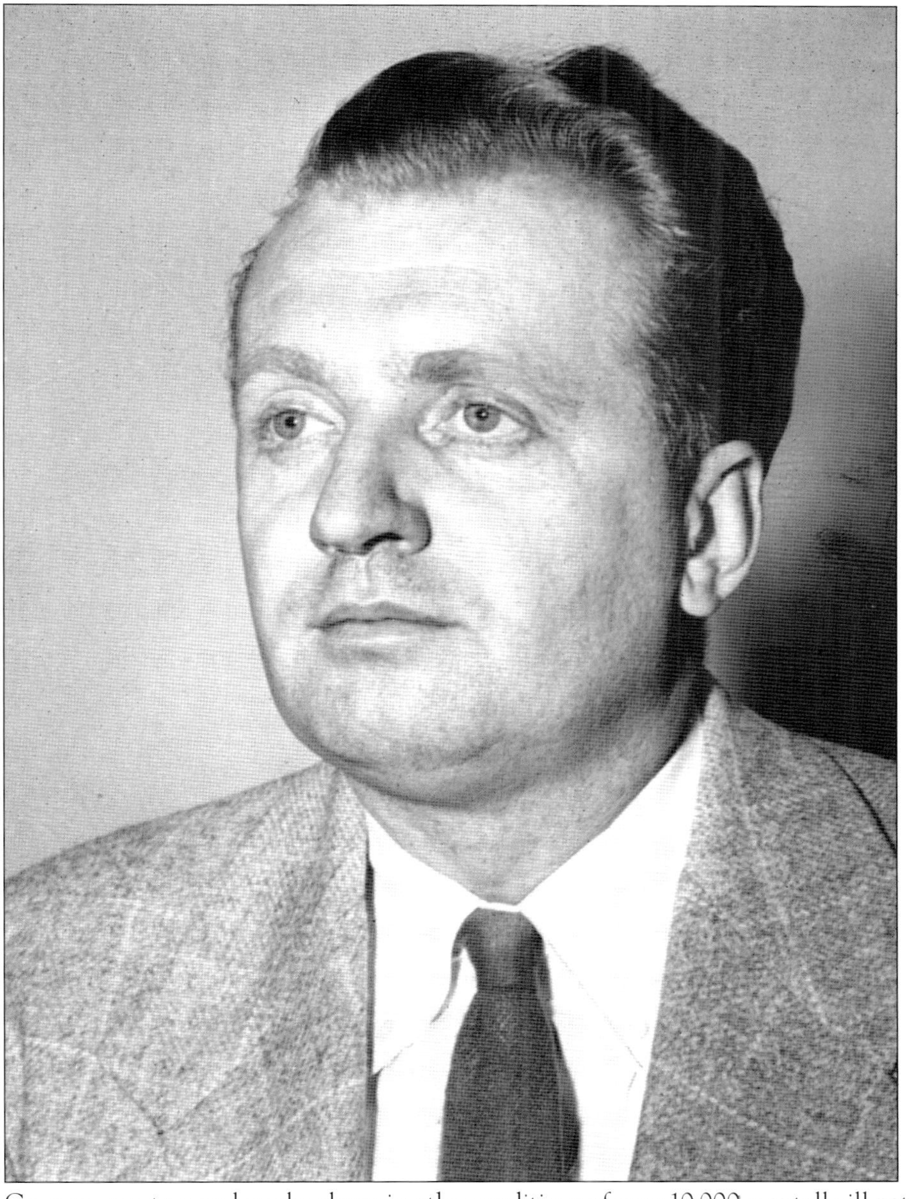

Mike Gorman spent several weeks observing the conditions of over 10,000 mentally ill patients in Oklahoma's state institutions. He described a "shameful story" of the "barbaric conditions under which the mentally ill lived." At first, Gorman did not want the story. He only initiated the investigation on the request of the bishop of Oklahoma City, who had a relative confined to one of the state hospitals. Gorman was apprehensive until he arrived in Norman. He got off the bus and walked along tree-lined streets with white frame houses toward the entrance of Central State Hospital and its grounds. He found the grounds well-groomed; it was like walking in a park. He waited in the administration building until superintendent Griffin joined him and escorted him to Hope Hall. It was here that Gorman began to understand the problem. "When the guard unlocked the big iron door and let us into the first ward," Gorman wrote, "an awful stench . . . hit me in the face." (OHS.)

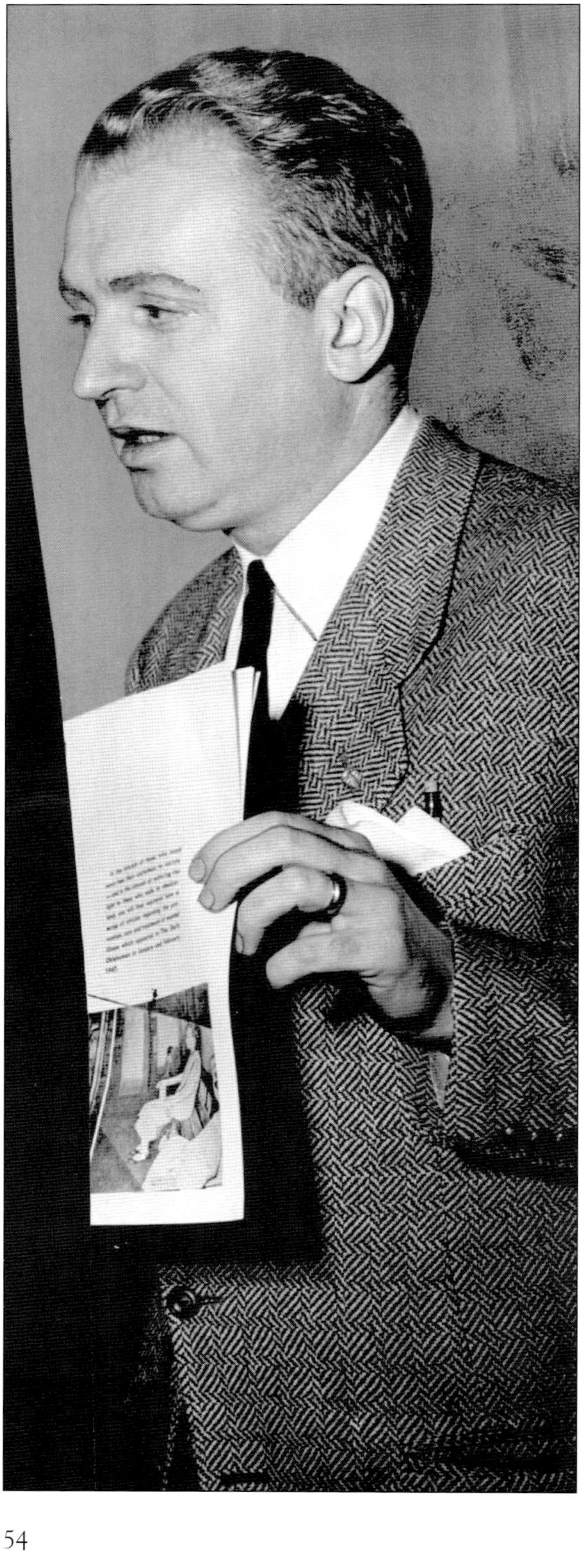

Gorman's investigative series, "Misery Rules in State Shadowland," ran in the *Daily Oklahoman* beginning in September 1946. Although Dr. Griffin, superintendent of Central State Hospital for 51 years, held advanced theories on how to cure the mentally ill and release them back into society, he lacked sufficient state appropriations to implement his programs. Gorman's observations in the *Daily Oklahoman* included "patients writhing and groveling on the floor; continued moaning and screaming; seclusion cells where patients, seen through peep-hole slits in the iron doors, thrashed about nakedly on cold stone floors." Gorman's exposé enlightened Oklahoma citizens about the problem and shamed state legislators into appropriating more money for state mental institutions. Unfortunately, Oklahoma's institutions were in line with others across the country. Gorman looked at past studies and wrote that a Brookings Institution study and the Oklahoma Planning and Resources Board recommendations described overcrowded and undermanned facilities and deplorable conditions for patients. (OHS.)

After his 1946 investigative report, Mike Gorman offered 10 recommendations that he believed should be implemented to change the apparent hopelessness of patients. The first and most obvious problem was overcrowding. In 1946, there were 2,844 patients crammed into wards that had a combined 2,200-bed capacity. Beds were tightly fitted together and had no side tables, and some patients had to step over other beds to get to their own sleeping area. (OHS.)

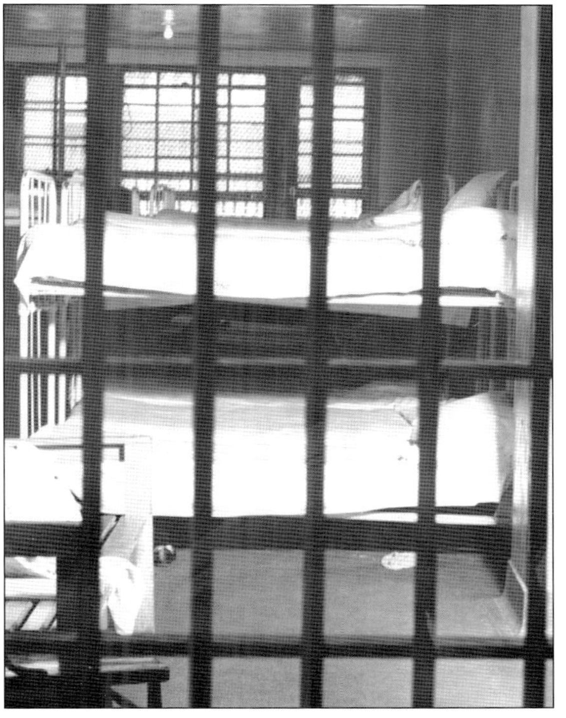

Another huge problem was the shortage of doctors. Even though the national standard recommended by the American National Psychiatric Institution was one doctor for every 150 patients, Oklahoma had one doctor for every 676 patients. There was also a shortage of nurses and attendants. In 1946, Oklahoma had seven graduate nurses, with five at Central State. The hospital also had only 89 regular attendants to oversee more than 2,800 patients. (OHS.)

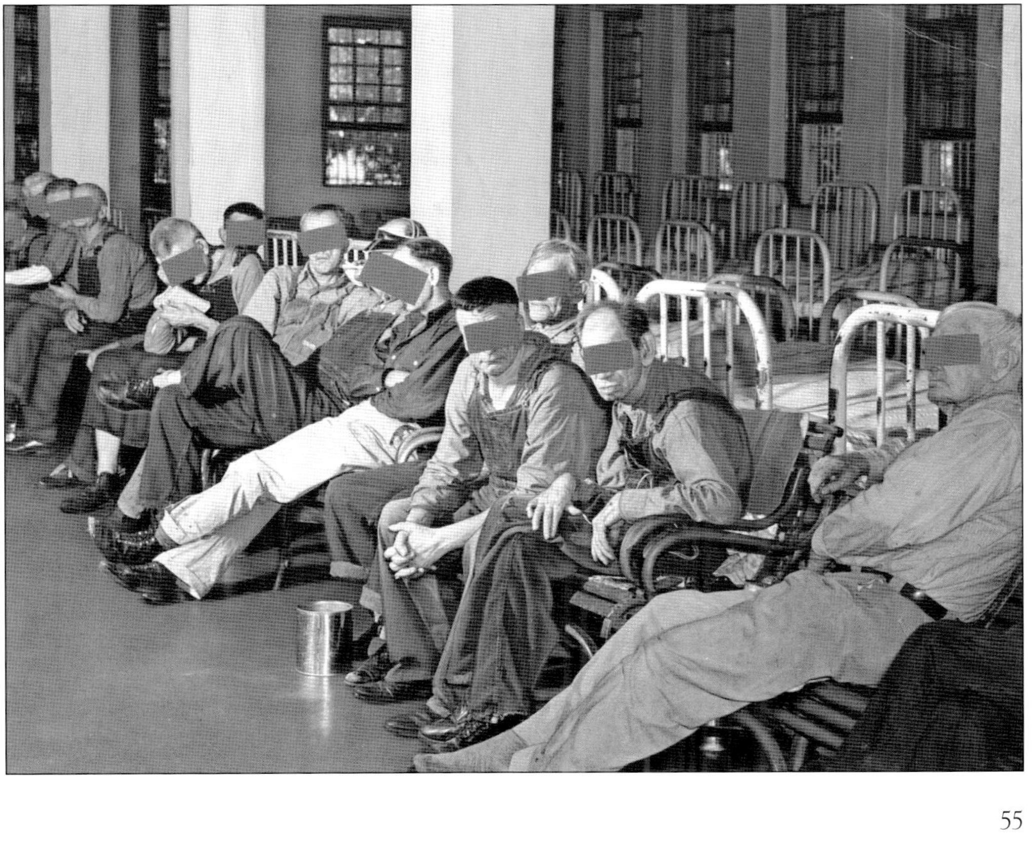

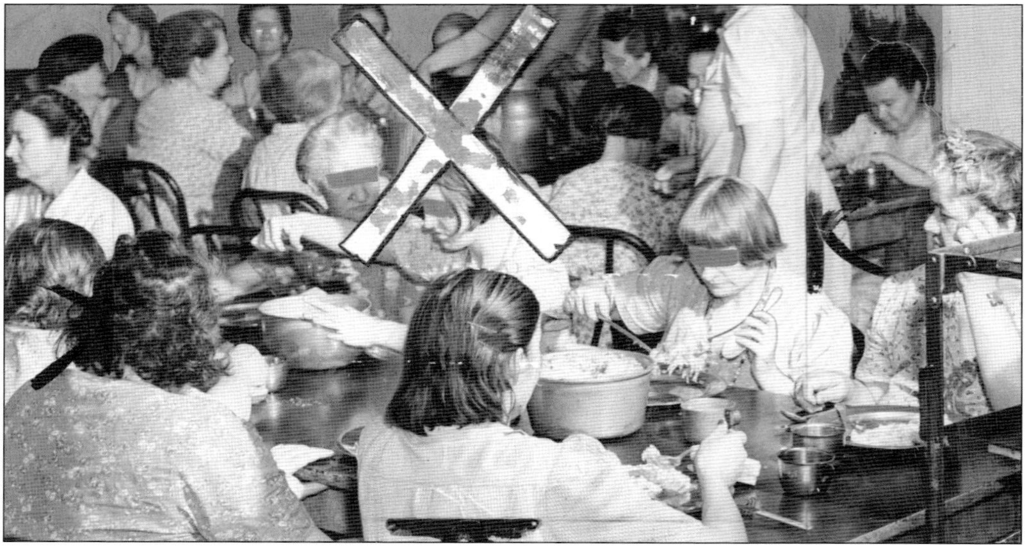

The dining hall on the first floor of Hope Hall was unsanitary and depressing. According to the 1946 articles by Mike Gorman, 50 patients pushed their way into the hall, where they sat at long wooden tables. An attendant brought the meals to the table in an aluminum pan and dumped a portion onto each patient's metal plate. (OHS.)

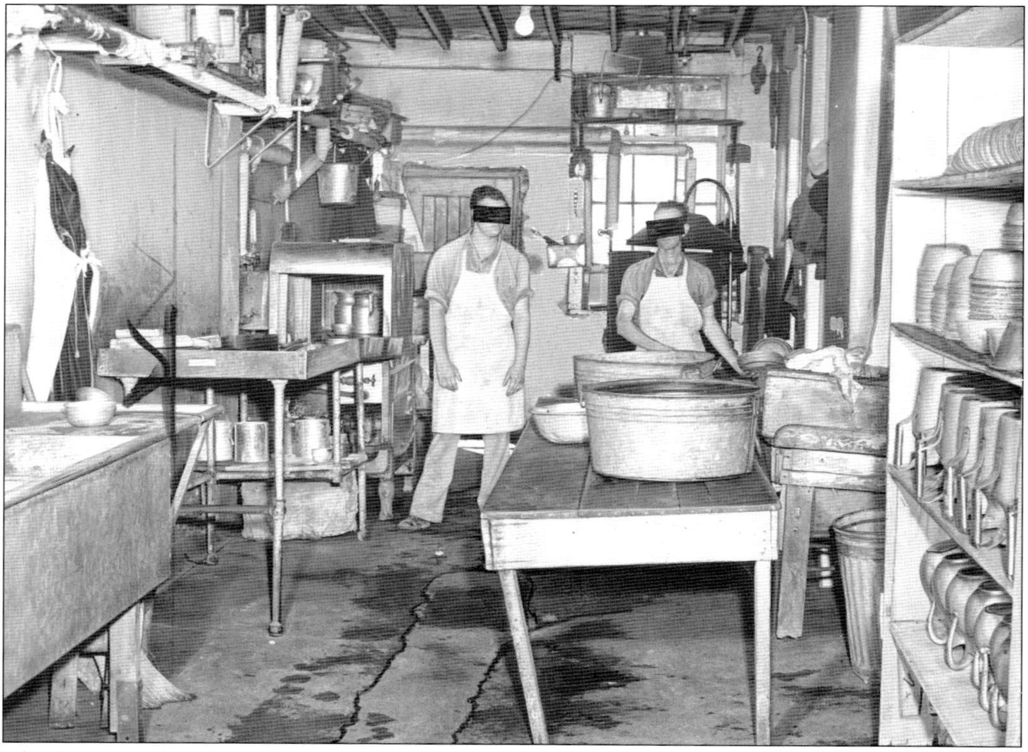

The kitchen where meals were prepared was indicative to Gorman of the general condition of the whole institution. Hopelessness and despair were also apparent in the wards, which had a lack of furniture, holes in the floors, large cracks in the walls, and unsanitary bathrooms. (OHS.)

Infrastructure such as that shown here pointed to the problem of maintaining Central State Hospital without appropriate funding. Most of the buildings suffered from a general lack of maintenance in addition to a terrible lack of sanitation. It was difficult for superintendent Griffin to administer treatment to patients in such an atmosphere. (OHS.)

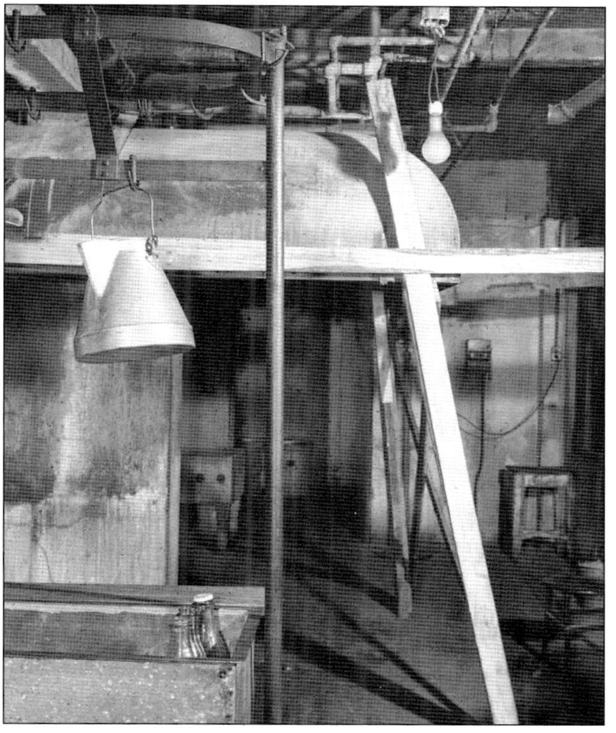

From the outside, Hope Hall looked like the institution that Dr. Griffin believed would offer hope and recovery to those in need. But the building itself could not offer hope; only the professional staff inside could give that to those who entered its evaluation center. Griffin continued to request more funding for professional staff, but to no avail. (OHS.)

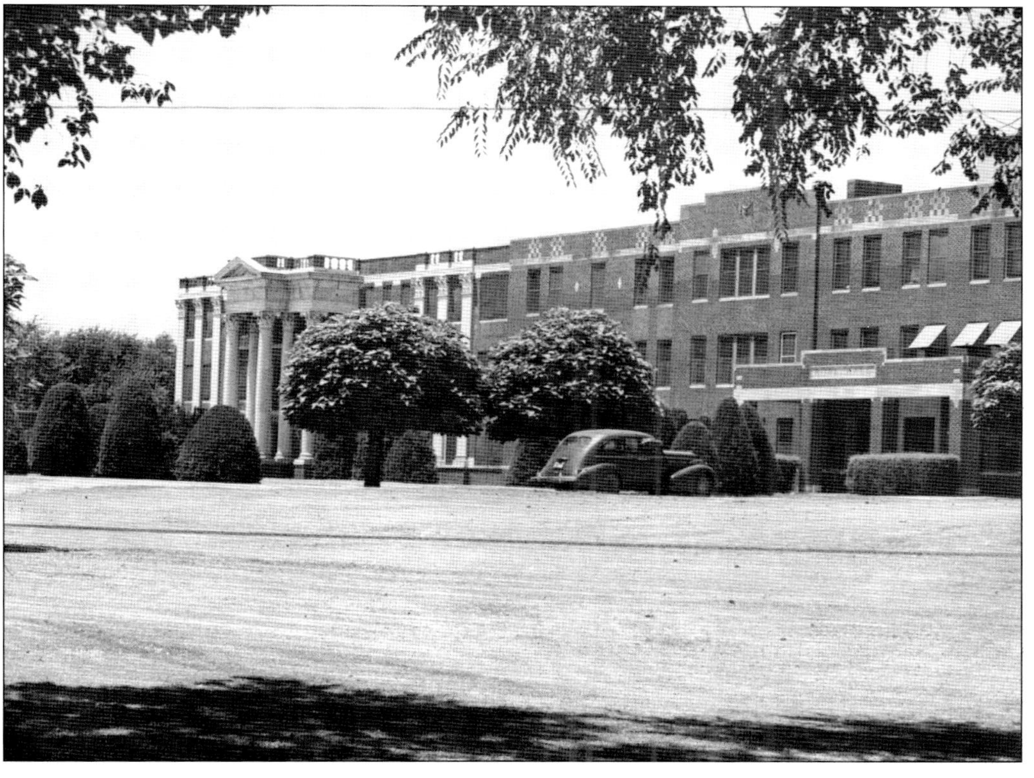

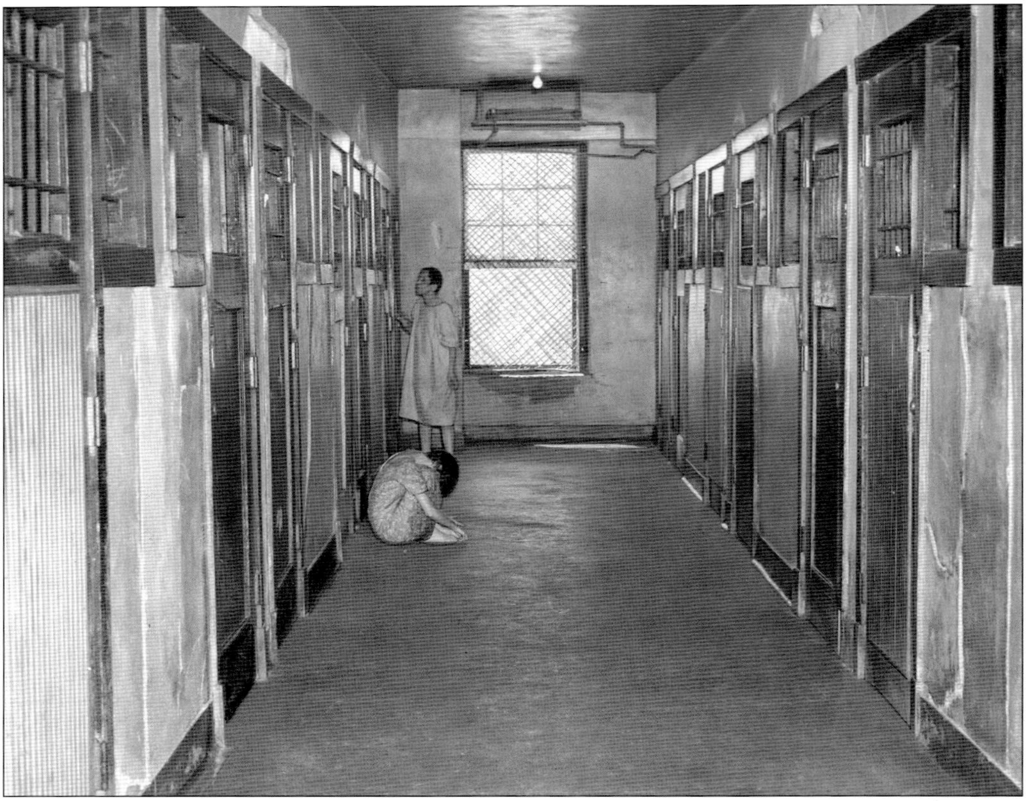

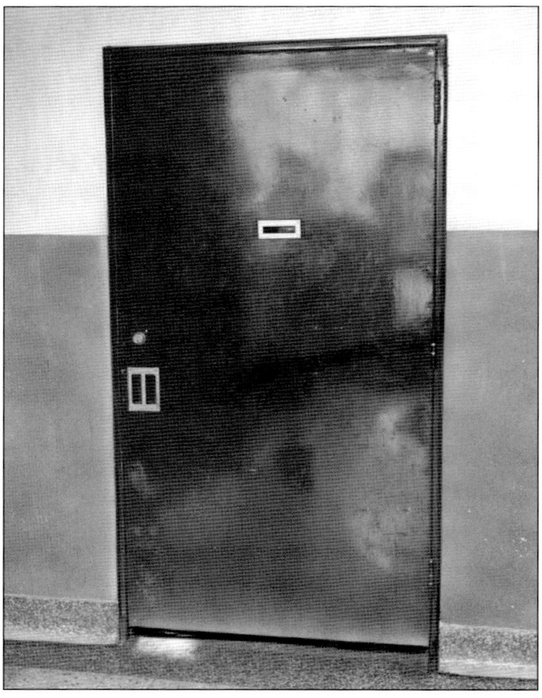

Overcrowded facilities and a lack of attendants made it almost impossible for Central State Hospital to treat minor mental conditions. Instead, all patients, regardless of their specific illnesses, were treated the same. Those who were diagnosed as violent were kept in seclusion cells for long periods of time, which violated modern psychiatric standards. Mike Gorman stated that on the second floor of Hope Hall, he could hear the screams of the women being kept in seclusion. (OHS.)

In the men's ward, the seclusion cells were like cages with a peephole in the door. There were no furnishings except a dirty mattress on the floor. The furnishings provided for the patients were wooden benches along the hallway walls. Gorman described the despair in the patients' attitudes and that most patients were not allowed outside their wards; a walk down the hall was a privilege. (OHS.)

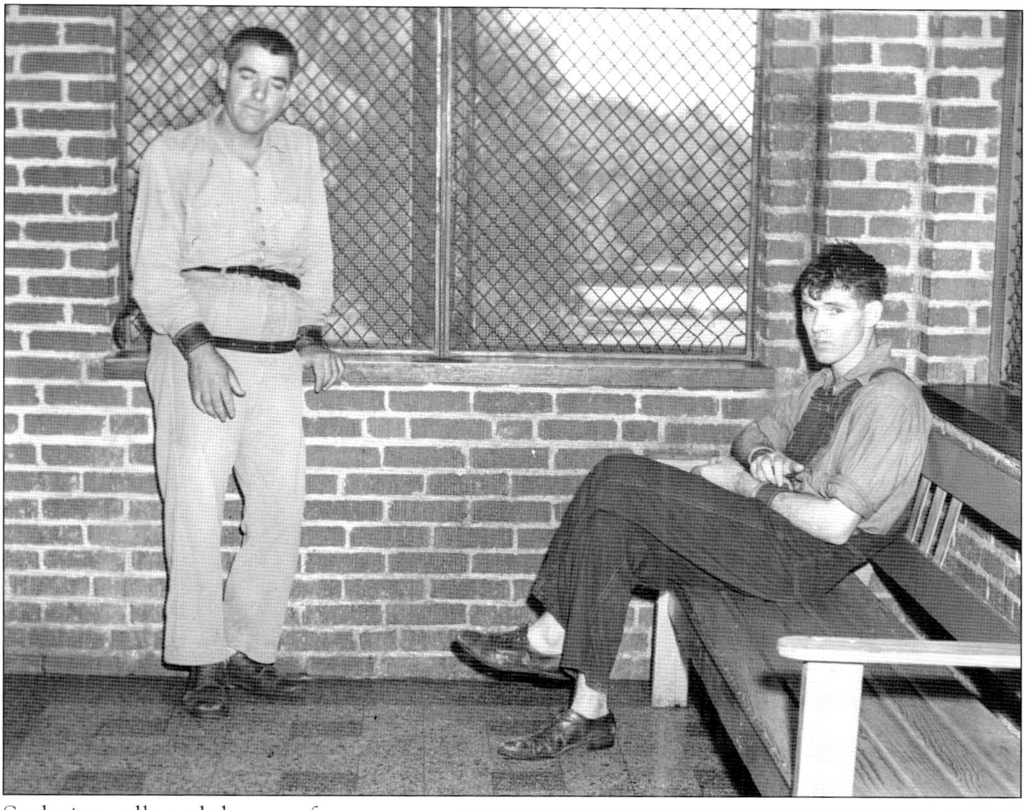

Seclusion cells and the use of restraints were not part of the national guidelines regarding psychiatric treatment in the 1940s, but with few doctors and attendants at Central State Hospital, restraints were often used to handle patients. Besides leather wristlets and belts, camisoles and restraining sheets were also used to control patients. (OHS.)

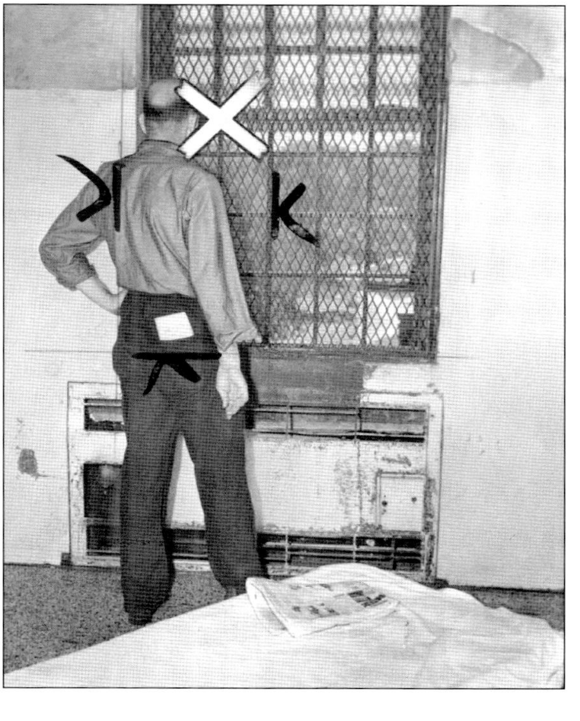

From Hope Hall, patients looked out of barred windows in despair. In the 1940s, different kinds of shock treatments were thought to be good therapy for those with acute mental illness. One idea was that large doses of insulin would "shock" a person back to normalcy. Although the treatments were costly, as Mike Gorman pointed out, they were less expensive than keeping patients under custodial care. (OHS.)

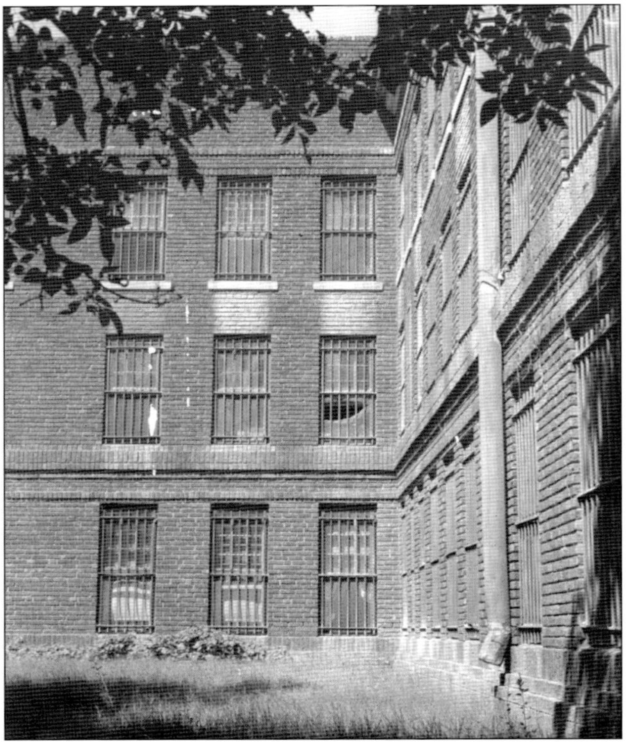

This picture of the back of Hope Hall offers a view of three stories of barred windows. If visitors were allowed on the grounds of Central State Hospital today, they would see that the bars still appear on many of the windows, a testament to the bleak world of those who sought treatment and were forced to view the world through bars.

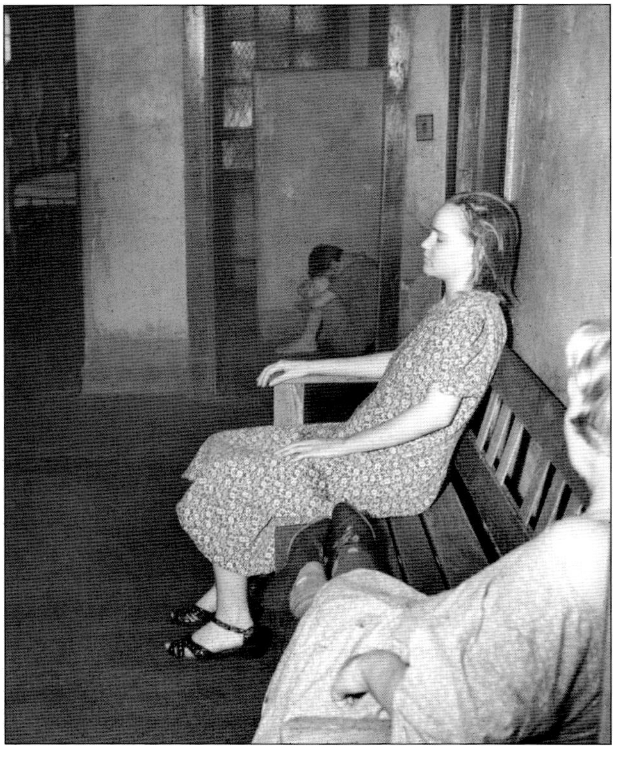

Electric shock, or electroconvulsive, therapy was another treatment used at Central State Hospital. According to the *Daily Oklahoman*, physicians believed that of the various treatments, electric shock was the most effective. The procedure involved applying probes to the frontal lobes of the brain. The treatment was sometimes successful in treating ailments that would be recognized today as depression, bipolar disorder, and schizophrenia. (OHS.)

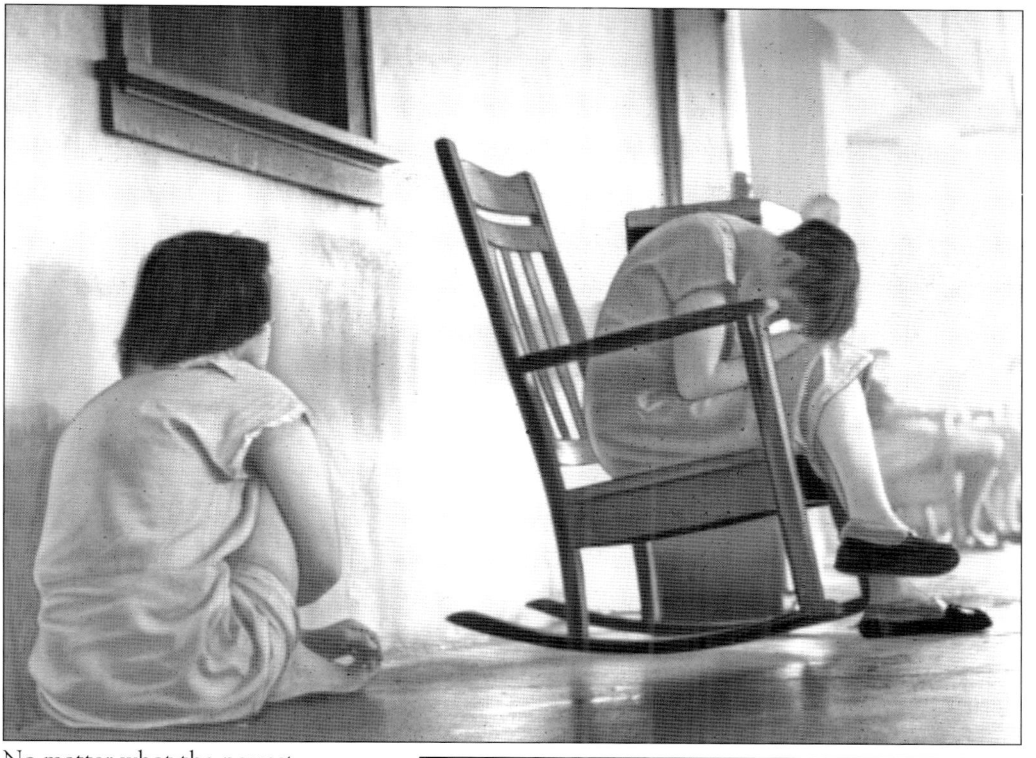

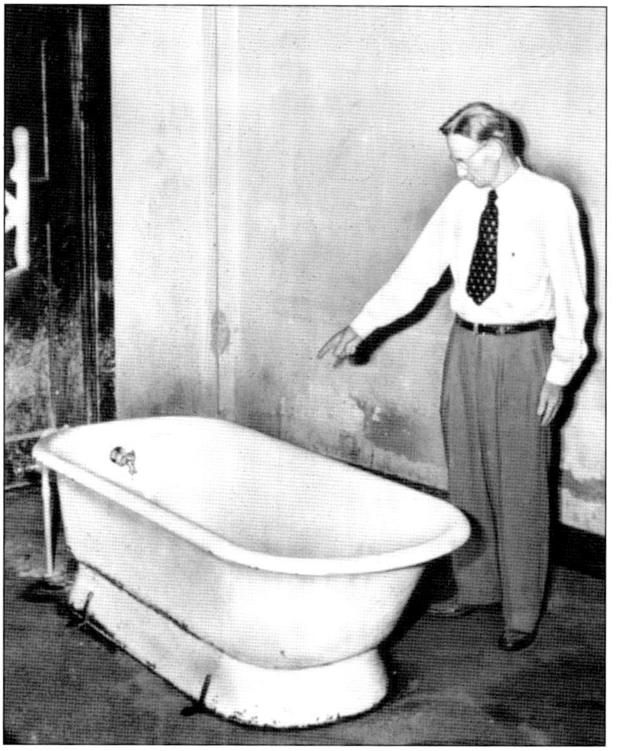

No matter what the newest treatment might be for acute and chronic mental cases, without experienced staff who could implement the treatments, many patients did not receive the treatment that was appropriate for them. Part of the problem of acquiring a trained medical staff was a lack of funding that would allow Oklahoma hospitals to compete in the national market for competent physicians. (OHS.)

Overcrowded conditions were visible in every aspect of life at Central State Hospital. This bathtub was the only bathing facility for 61 women in 1949. In the lavatory, according to Mike Gorman, was a "chamber of horrors" where dirty toilets had no curtains or walls. (OHS.)

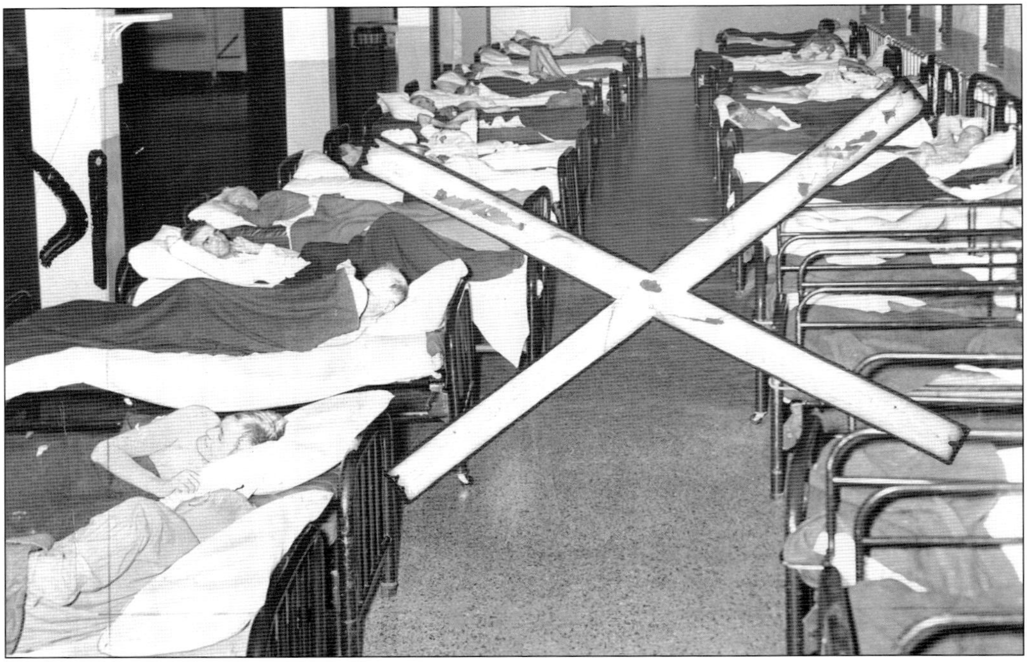

The overcrowded wards and lack of attendants that Mike Gorman outlined in his *Daily Oklahoman* articles highlighted conditions that led to the abuse of patients. This picture accompanied an article in the *Norman Transcript* about attendants beating patients in the crowded ward. (OHS.)

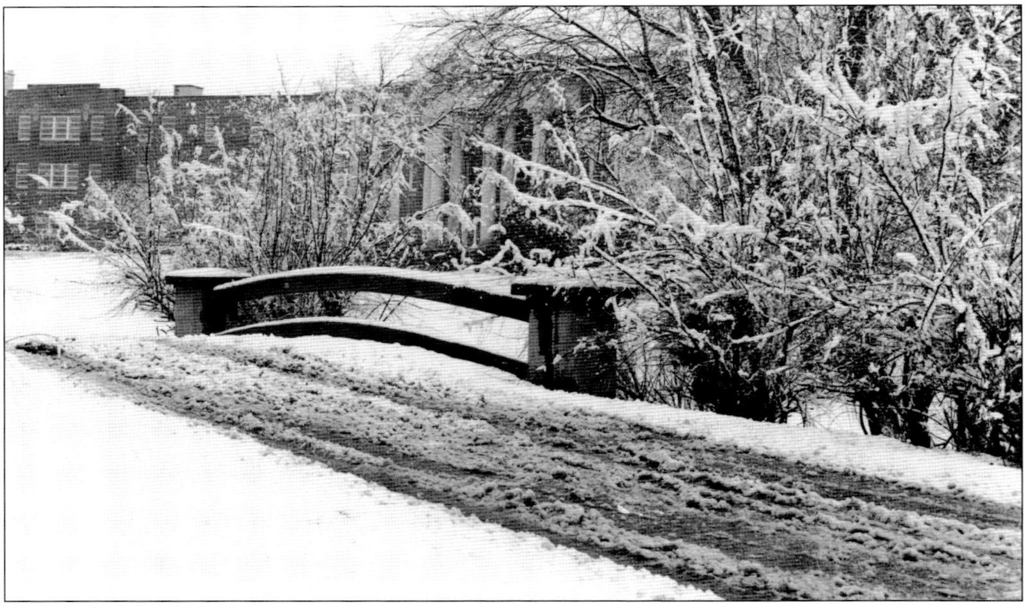

Regardless of state appropriations for new wards at Central State Hospital, there still was not enough money or professional personnel to improve the conditions inside the wards. There was an ongoing cycle of building wards to house more patients, which in turn created more overcrowding. The result of insufficient funds to keep up with crowded conditions and insufficient programs became more investigations into the conditions at state hospitals. (OHS.)

In the 1940s, the veterans' building at Central State Hospital held 225 mentally ill veterans from both world wars; it was an exception to the terrible conditions of the other wards. The state legislature continued to provide sufficient funds for disabled veterans, which provided for more modern facilities. (OHS.)

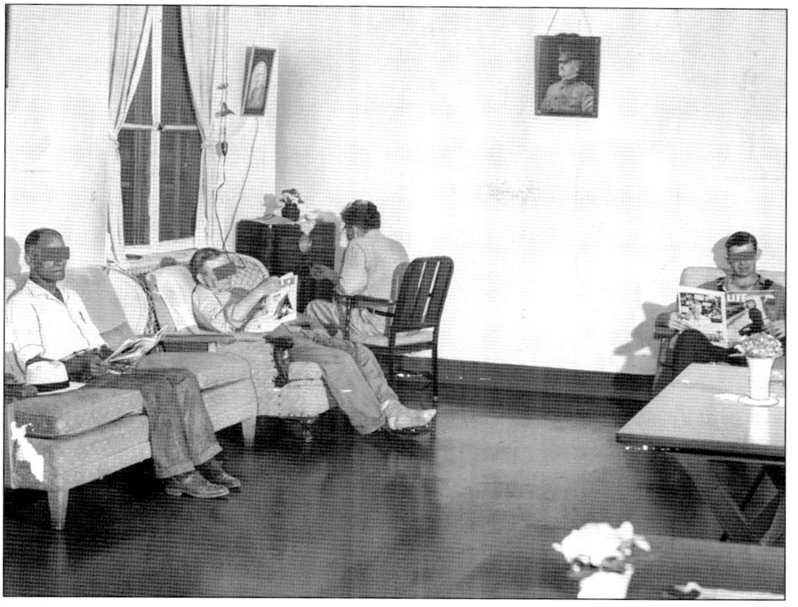

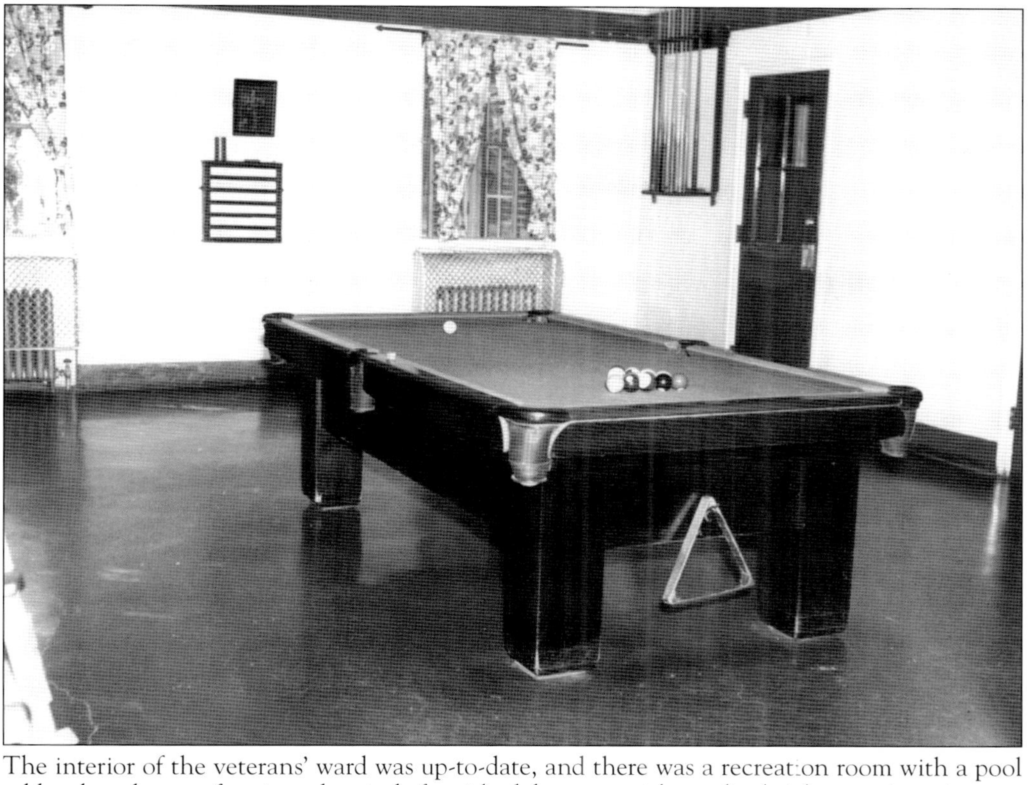

The interior of the veterans' ward was up-to-date, and there was a recreation room with a pool table, plus a large cafeteria and a nicely furnished dayroom with a radio, bright curtains, pictures, and fresh paint. Since World War I, superintendent Griffin had believed that veterans who suffered shell shock and other mental trauma could be brought back to normal mental health if they were treated separately from other mental patients. (OHS.)

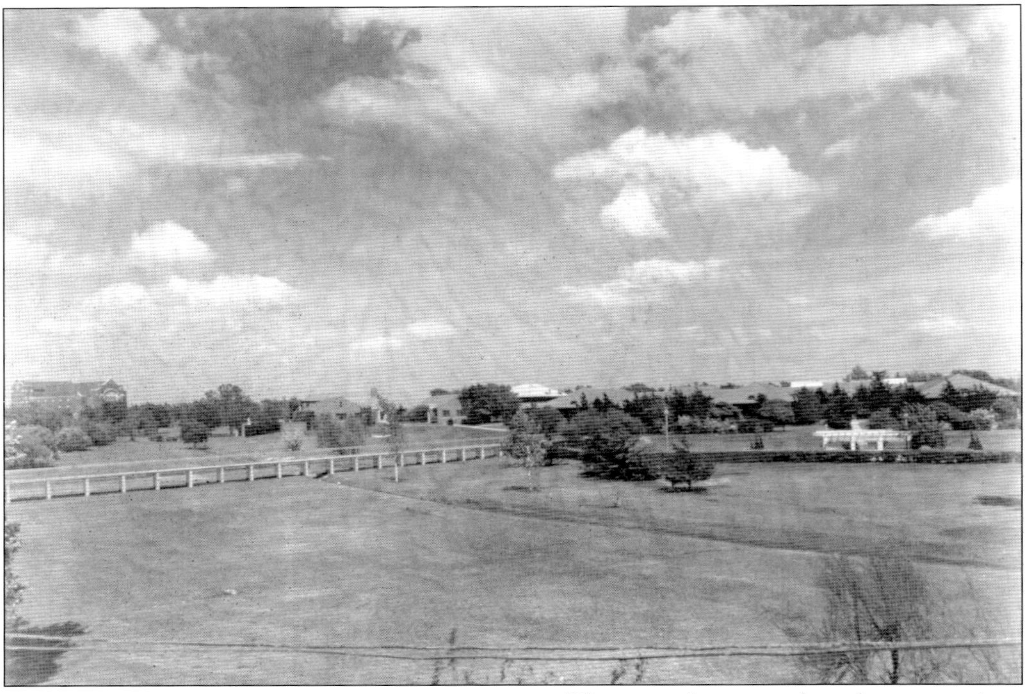

The grounds surrounding the veterans' buildings at Central State Hospital were maintained to provide a parklike atmosphere, which was considered good for the mental well-being of the veterans. This image shows a rose arbor and garden outside the veterans' wards. (CCHS.)

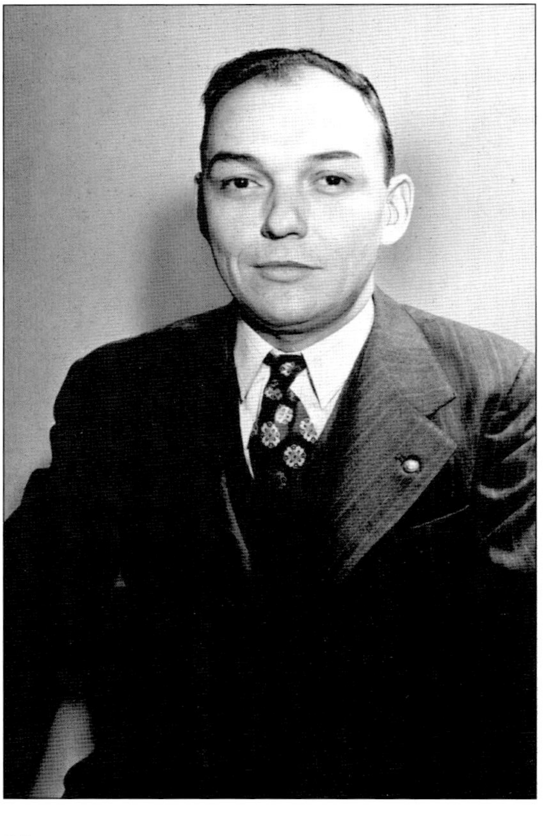

In 1949, Oklahoma state representative Robert O. Cunningham of Oklahoma County led the fight in the state legislature for appropriations to improve the deteriorating conditions inside state mental institutions. Cunningham described conditions as "one big, horrible mess with the patients receiving the little end of the deal." The legislature appropriated more funds for new buildings and funds to remodel existing wards. (OHS.)

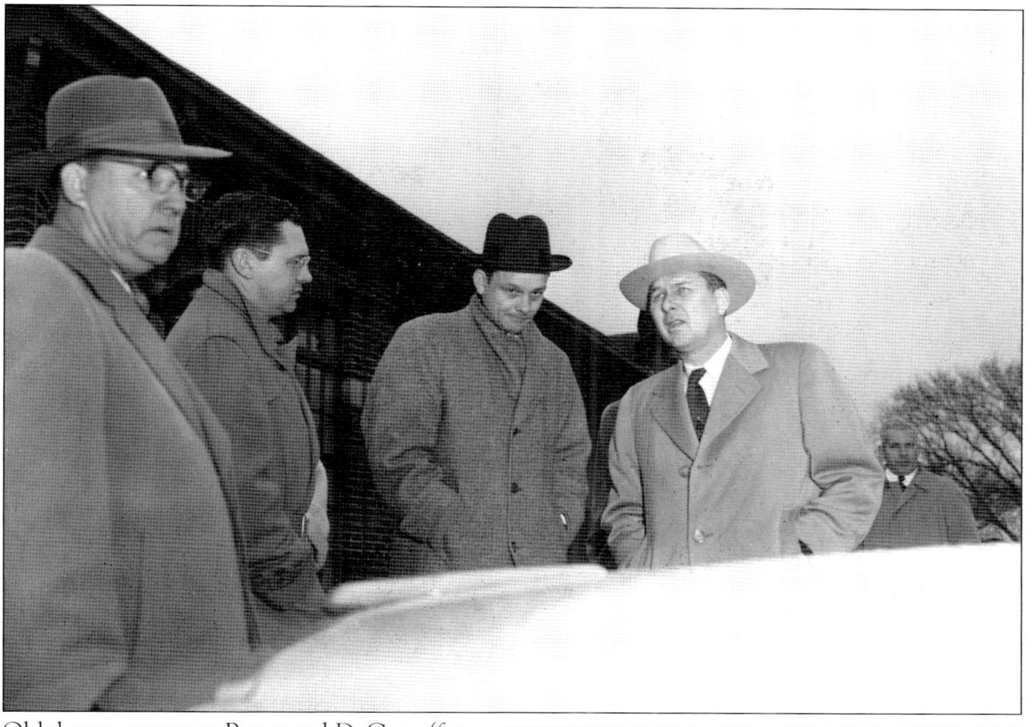

Oklahoma governor Raymond D. Gary (far right) inspected Central State Hospital in 1955. Gary was trying to decide whether a legislative proposal for a three-man board to oversee 21 state institutions would be sufficient. He believed that there should be a seven-man team on the committee and that the decision to form the oversight committee should be put to the voters in the next election. (OHS.)

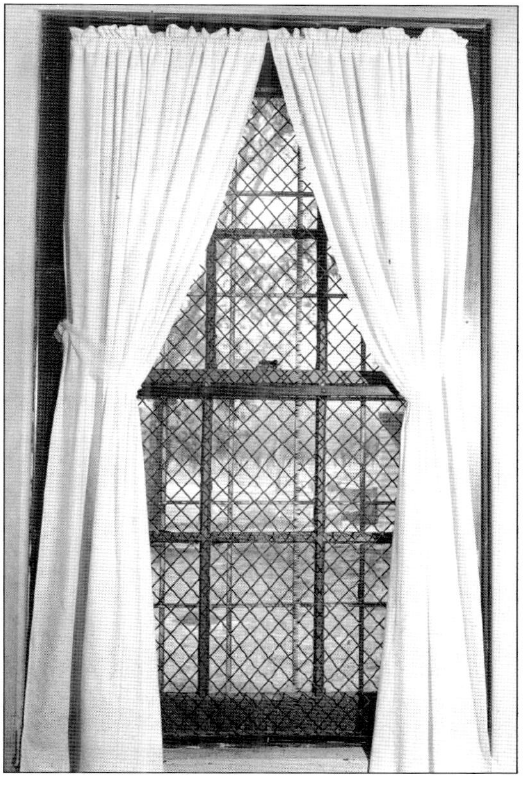

The 1950s marked a turning point at Central State Hospital. Some barred windows gave way to safety windows without bars, which changed the atmosphere of hopelessness that may have contributed to deterring doctors and staff from providing an environment conducive to the well-being of the patients. The change was a result of the investigations that had created public outcry and prompted more legislative appropriations. (OHS.)

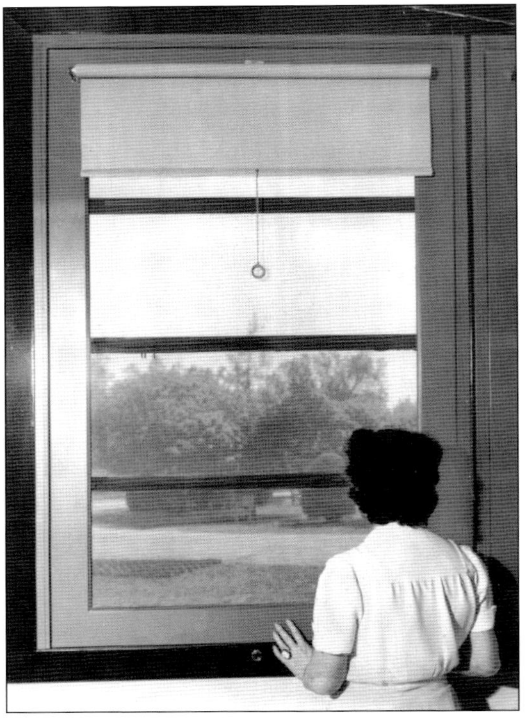

The new buildings constructed at Central State Hospital after the investigations were designed to offer more light by providing more windows. The new windows were casement windows equipped with detention screens. These windows were reported to be escape-proof, which theoretically made it impossible for disturbed patients to break the glass. (OHS.)

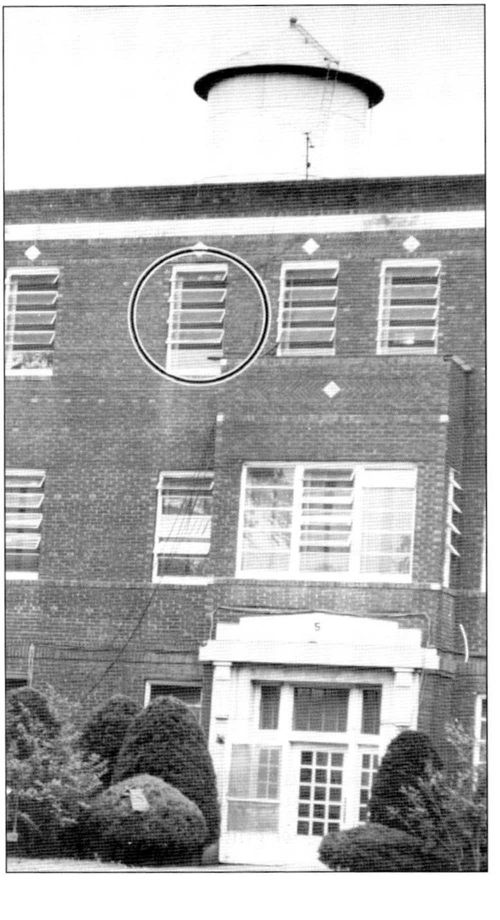

Regardless of how "escape-proof" the windows were supposed to be, Harley Ed Dickerson escaped from the third floor of a maximum-security ward at Central State Hospital between 2:00 a.m. and 5:30 a.m. one day in April 1969. Dickerson, who was at Central State while awaiting trial for two counts of murder, worked loose a bar on a window, bent the bar away from the steel screen, and pulled back the screen. He then tied blankets together and lowered himself to the ground. (OHS.)

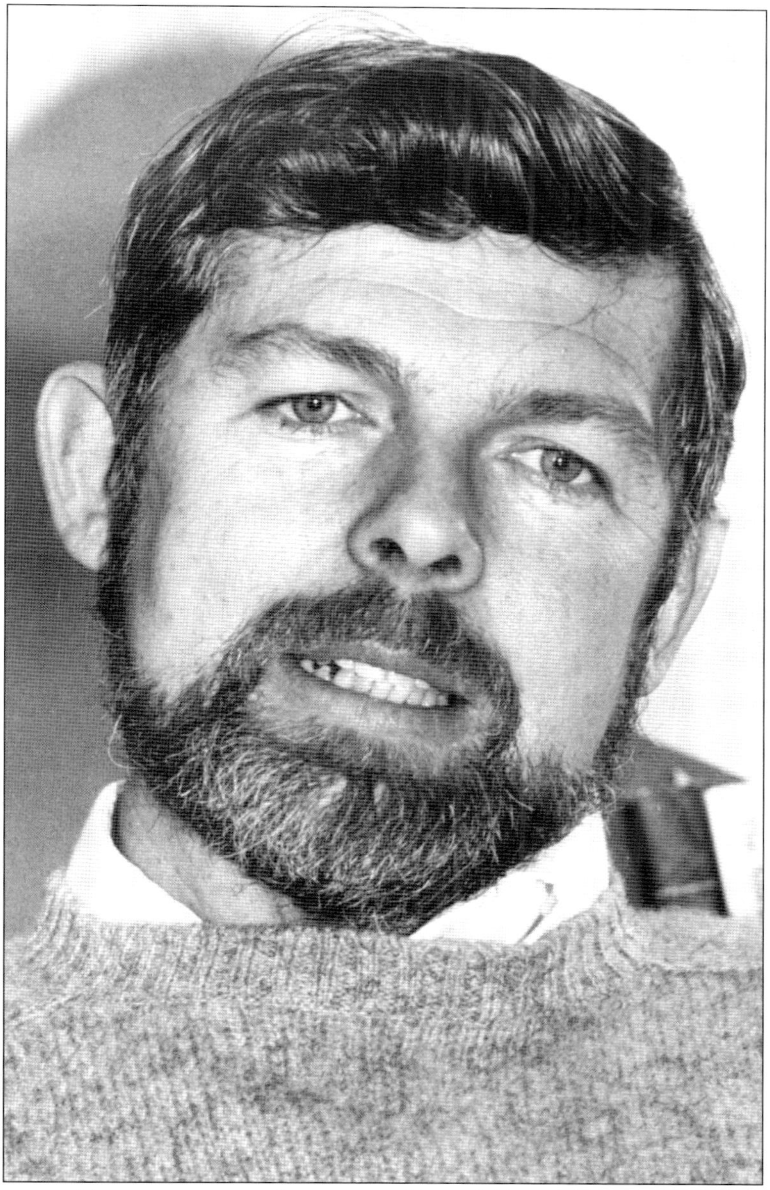

Trouble with unstable patients was a frequent problem. Well into the 1980s, patients still acted out against staff members at Central State Hospital. In August 1987, a mental health aide was beaten by one of the patients. The incident caused many to be concerned about the security at Central State. In the fall of 1987, patient advocate Larry Siria, seen here, was shot by one of his former patients. Siria, a graduate of the University of Oklahoma School of Law, was shot while sitting at his desk in the administration building. One of Siria's former patients was arrested for the shooting. Siria was taken to Norman Regional Hospital. After two weeks, he was released from the hospital with the bullet still in his back. Two weeks later, he died of a pulmonary embolism as a result of the shooting. The Oklahoma Department of Mental Health formed a task force to recommend tougher guidelines and to educate professionals about how to deal with aggressive patients. (OHS.)

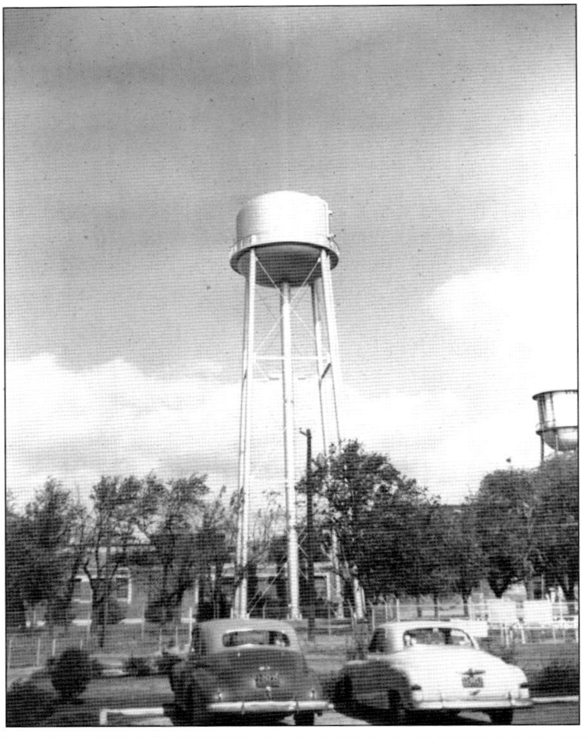

Understaffing and overcrowding resulted in fewer patient attendants. It was not uncommon for disturbed and unhappy patients to find ways to escape their misery. Some tried to escape like Harley Ed Dickerson (see page 66), who was pursued by police in a manhunt around the hospital grounds and throughout Cleveland County. Others attempted suicide. This tower was used by a patient who committed suicide by jumping from it. (OHS.)

A $1.5 million state appropriation to Central State Hospital in 1950 provided the hospital with 300 more beds for tuberculosis patients, which opened space in other wards to help alleviate overcrowding. Overcrowding and a lack of physical space for patients was an ongoing problem, but in the 1950s, the Oklahoma legislature began to supply enough funds to finally make a difference. (OHS.)

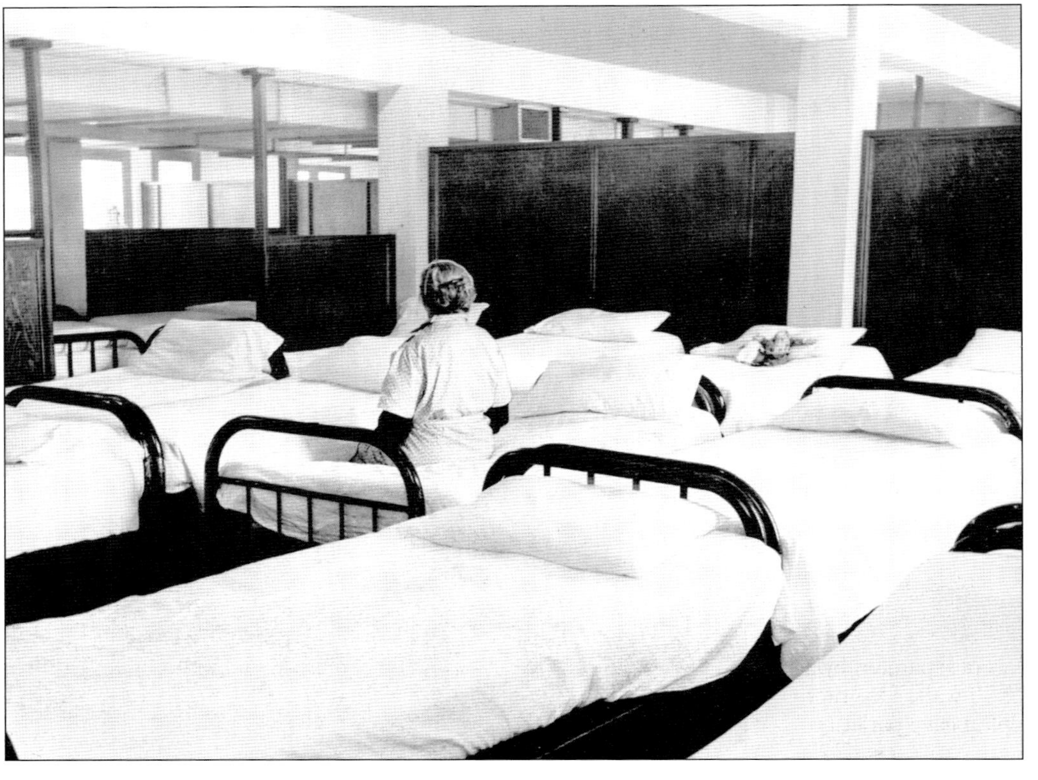

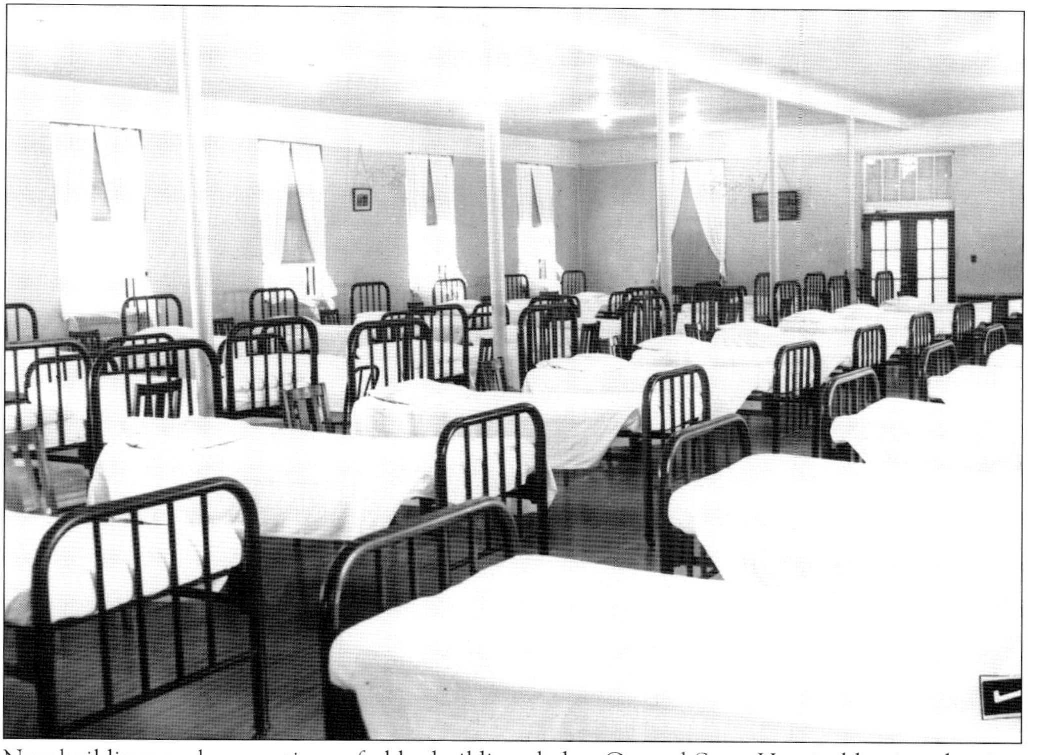

New buildings and renovations of older buildings led to Central State Hospital having sleeping wards with space between the beds, and each patient had a chair next to their bed. The celebrated Hope Hall and its two annexes received extensive remodeling, which included new plumbing and heating. The old radiators were a constant hazard to the patients. (OHS.)

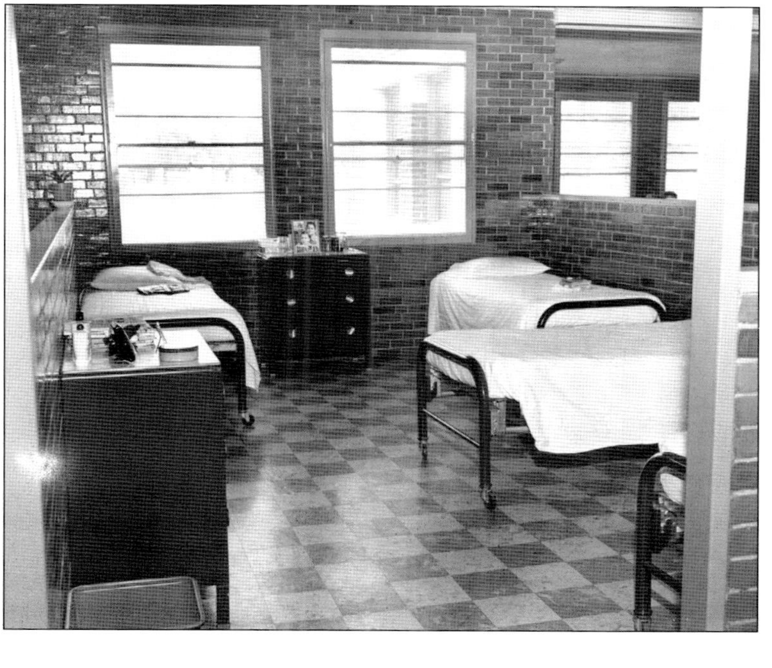

One wing of Hope Hall that previously held disturbed female patients and had beds that were crammed together was renovated to include partitioned sleeping areas. Each section held four beds that were separated by a half wall. This new plan gave patients more privacy. (OHS.)

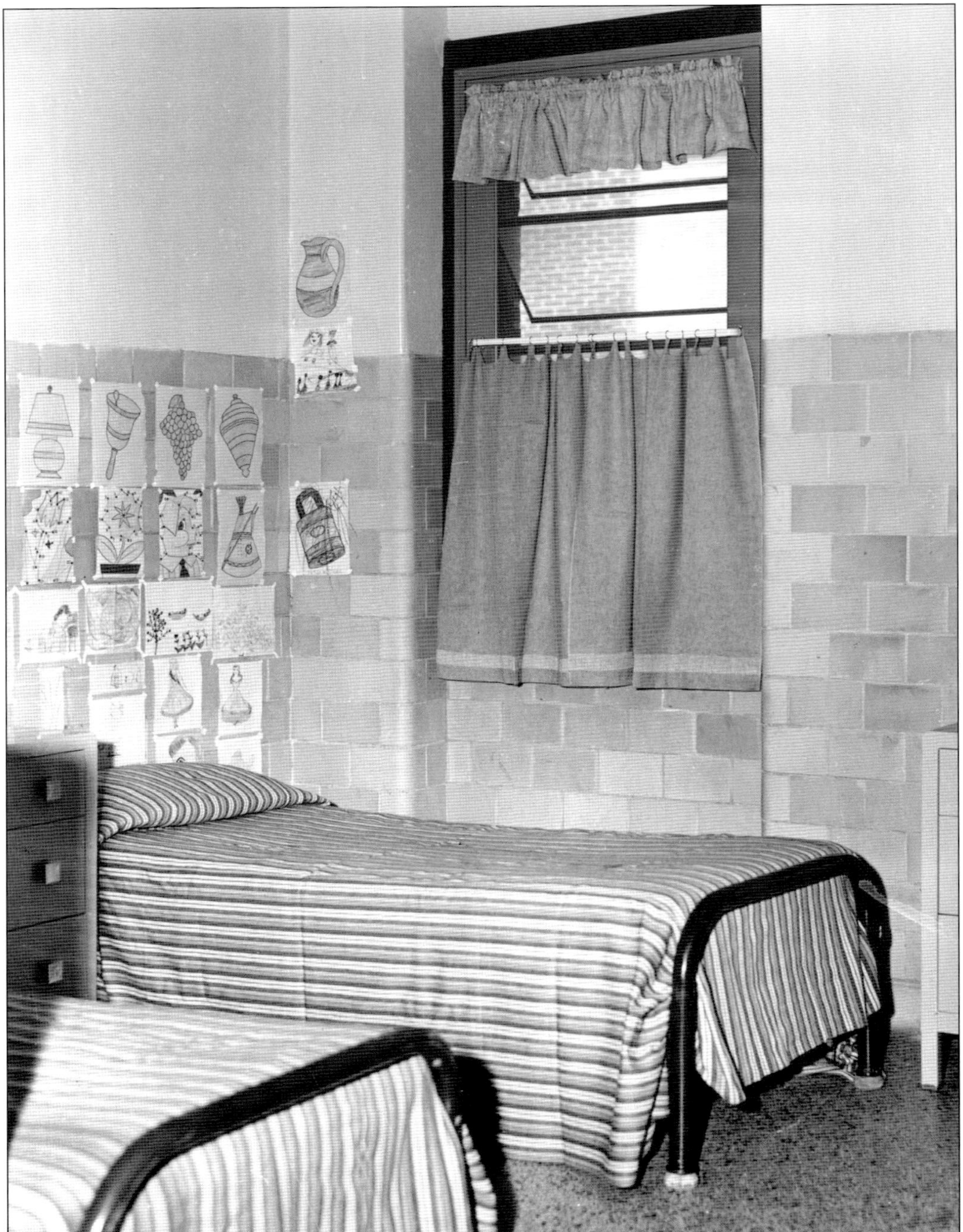

Also in the 1950s, more attention was paid to children and young adults who resided at Central State Hospital. As with the renovated women's wards, the new children's wards were less crowded and more private than in the preceding decade. Girls from sororities at the University of Oklahoma, members of various Girl Scout troops, and Camp Fire Girls provided programs and parties in the children's wards for Valentine's Day and Christmas. (OHS.)

Four

A New Era
1950s

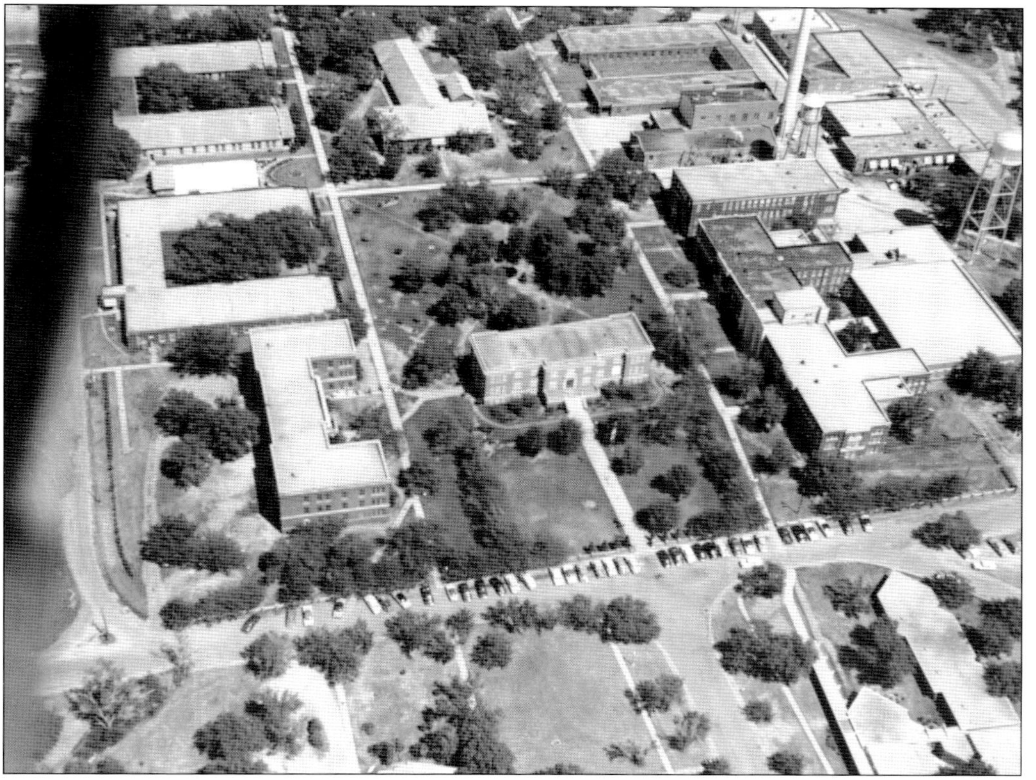

The 1950s ushered in a new era at Central State Hospital. The investigations of the 1940s resulted in significant state appropriations to alleviate overcrowding, but perhaps just as important were funding programs that helped patients to fully recover. There was also a turnover in administration. After 51 years at the hospital, Dr. David Griffin retired in 1950, and in 1961, Dr. Hayden H. Donahue was appointed superintendent. (OHS.)

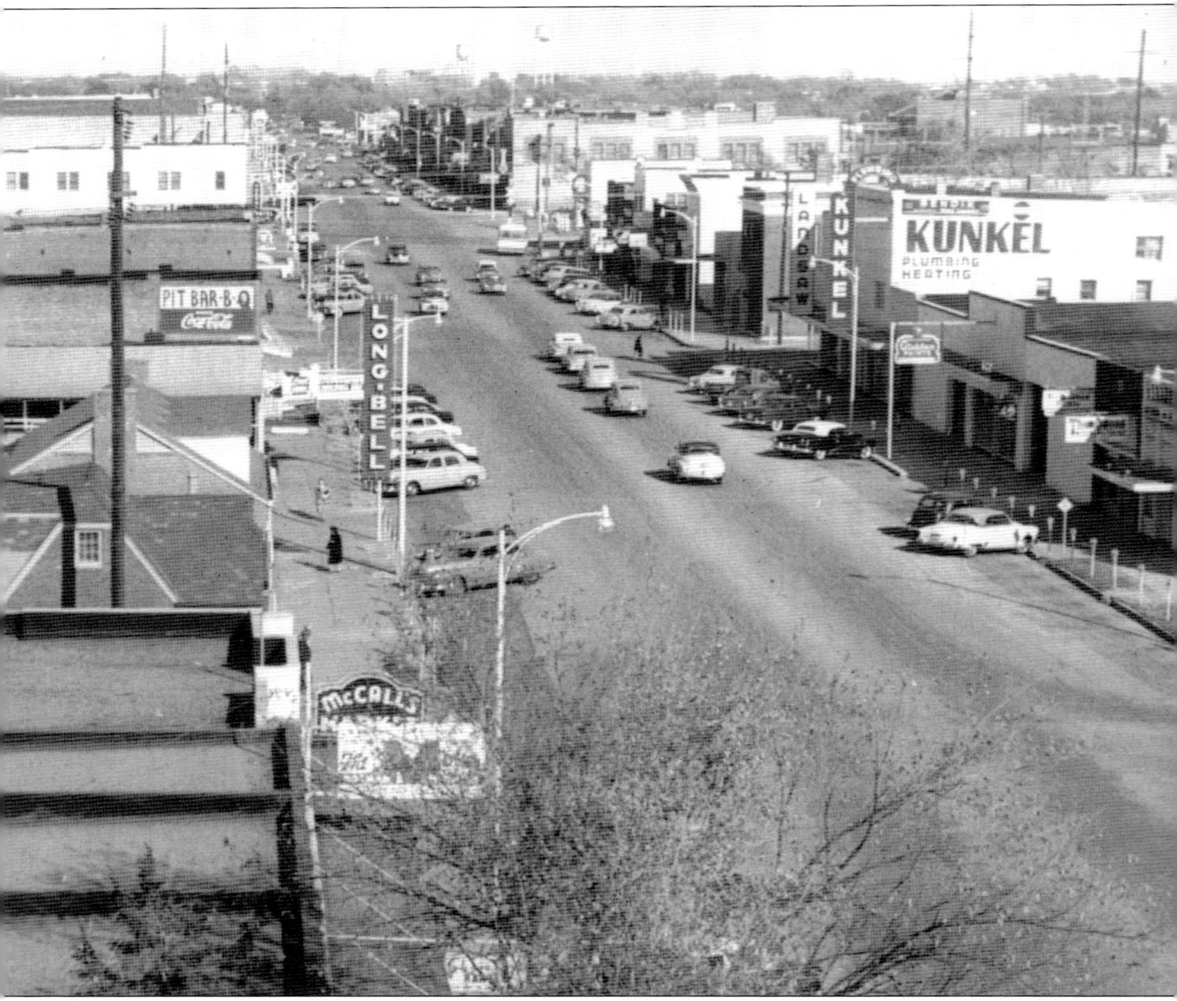

Both the City of Norman and Central State Hospital suffered financially in the Great Depression. For Central State, during the 1930s and 1940s, state funding all but dried up. In the 1940s, state financial resources were allocated for economic recovery and for the state's share of financing World War II. The 1950s brought economic changes to Norman and Central State; Norman had benefitted economically from the two Navy bases, and investigations into Oklahoma's mental hospitals in the 1940s increased the public's recognition of mental illness. Public pressure was on the state legislature to increase appropriations for the state's mental institutions. In the 1950s, with additional appropriations for new buildings and more funds to hire physicians, attendants, and nurses, a new era began in treatment for the mentally ill in Oklahoma. (CCHS.)

Dr. David Griffin began working at the Oklahoma Sanitarium Company in 1899. He watched it become a self-contained mental hospital while fighting for more money to improve conditions and treatment for patients. His legacy was in his work to educate the public that mental disorders deserved the same amount of money and treatment that was afforded to those with physical illnesses. (OHS.)

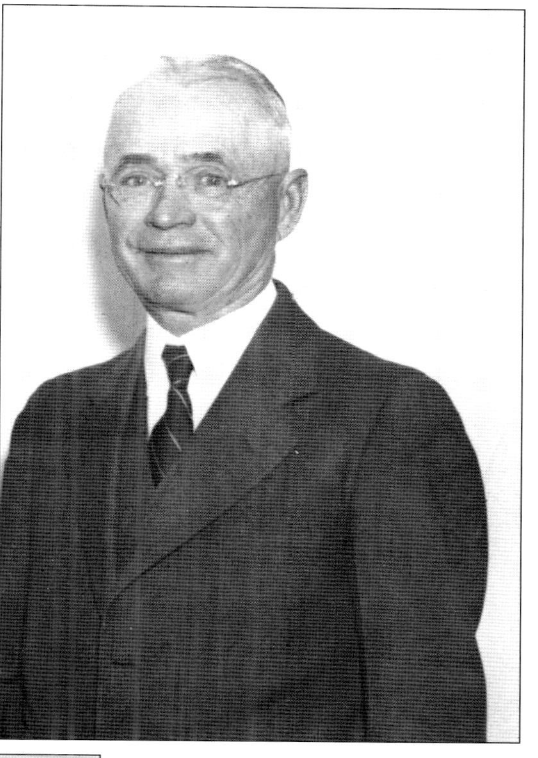

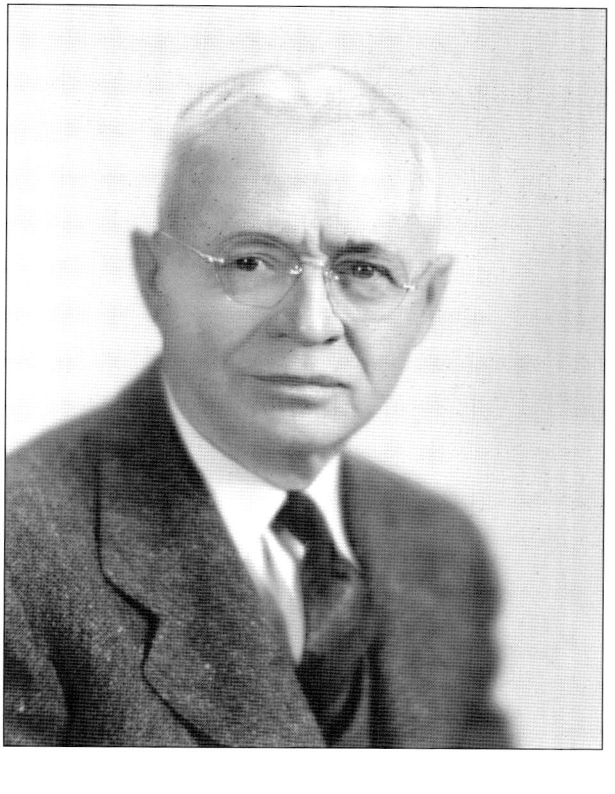

Dr. Griffin retired from Central State Hospital in 1950. During his tenure as superintendent, he fought many battles. One was to provide hospitals for shell-shocked veterans returning home from war. These men were assigned to asylums with patients whose mental illnesses were of a different nature. Griffin recognized this and fought for separate veterans' facilities at Central State. (OHS.)

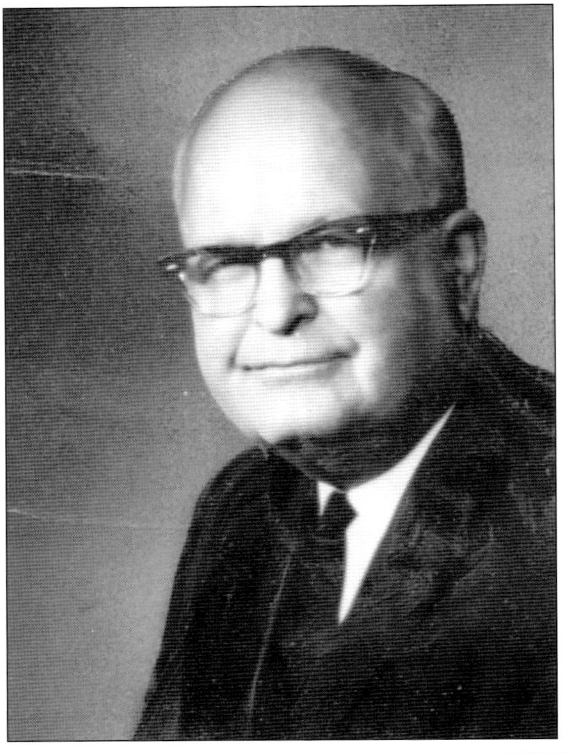

Dr. Charles A. Smith was one of four administrators at Central State Hospital in the 1950s. Smith was the first to succeed Griffin. His tenure as superintendent was met with accusations and investigations from the state legislature. The investigative committee reported that there were some staff members at Central State with alcohol problems and attendants who frequently beat the patients. The legislature asked Smith to resign, and he did so in July 1953. (OHS.)

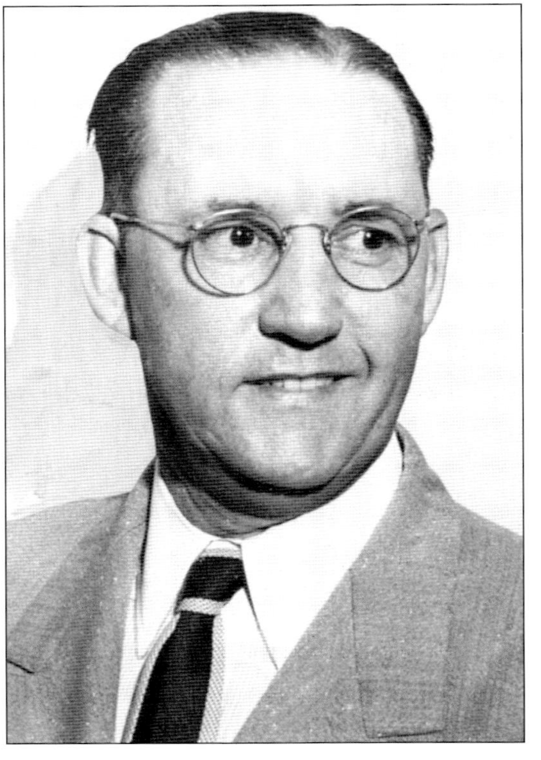

Dr. H.B. Whitten succeeded Dr. Smith as superintendent in 1953. The 46-year-old Whitten was a native of Gotebo, Oklahoma, where he practiced general medicine. After his service in the Army during World War II, he studied neuropsychiatry. The Oklahoma Board of Health praised Whitten for his philosophy that recognized the human dignity of mental patients. (OHS.)

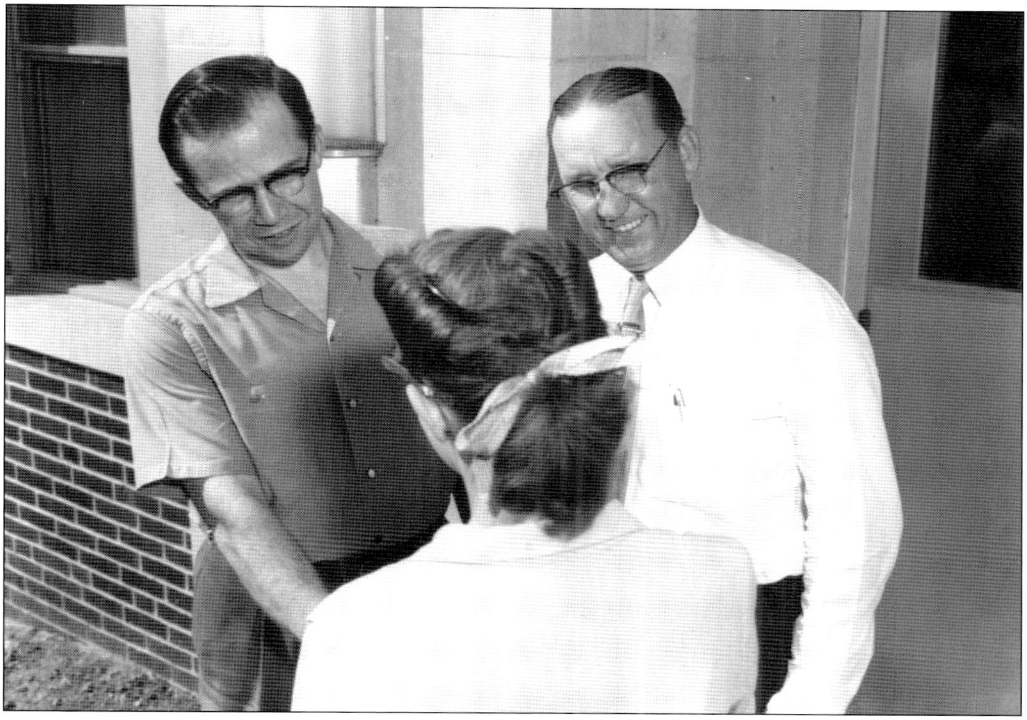

In 1956, the Oklahoma Board of Health appointed Dr. H.G. Hightower (left) as superintendent of Central State Hospital. In 1950, Hightower was the director of the Kiowa County Health Department. In 1952, he served as a neurologist at the Menninger Hospital in Topeka, Kansas. Hightower received his medical degree from the University of Oklahoma. (OHS.)

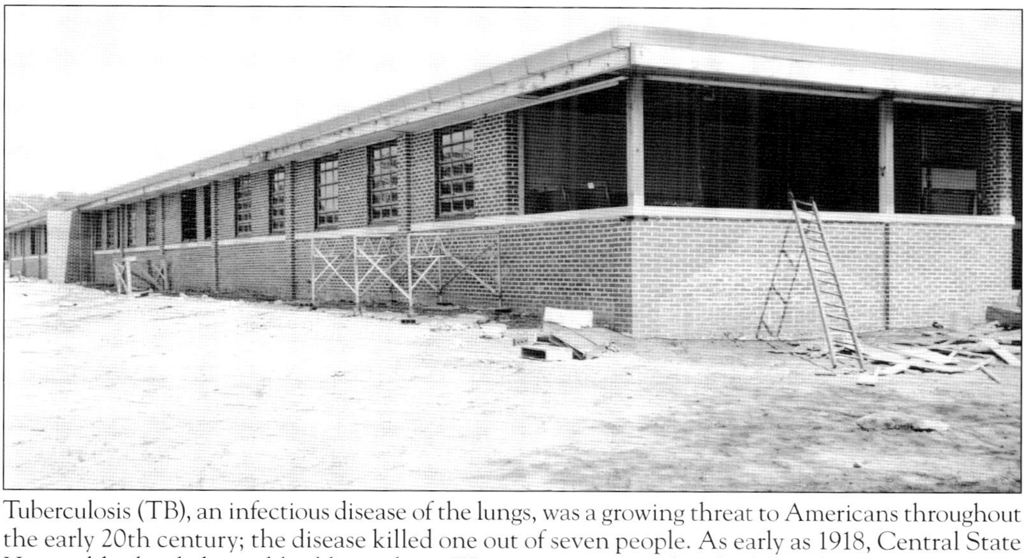

Tuberculosis (TB), an infectious disease of the lungs, was a growing threat to Americans throughout the early 20th century; the disease killed one out of seven people. As early as 1918, Central State Hospital had a dedicated building where TB patients were isolated, although the state did not recognize Central State as an official TB sanitarium. In the 1950s, new construction began on a TB ward (pictured) at Central State. (CCHS.)

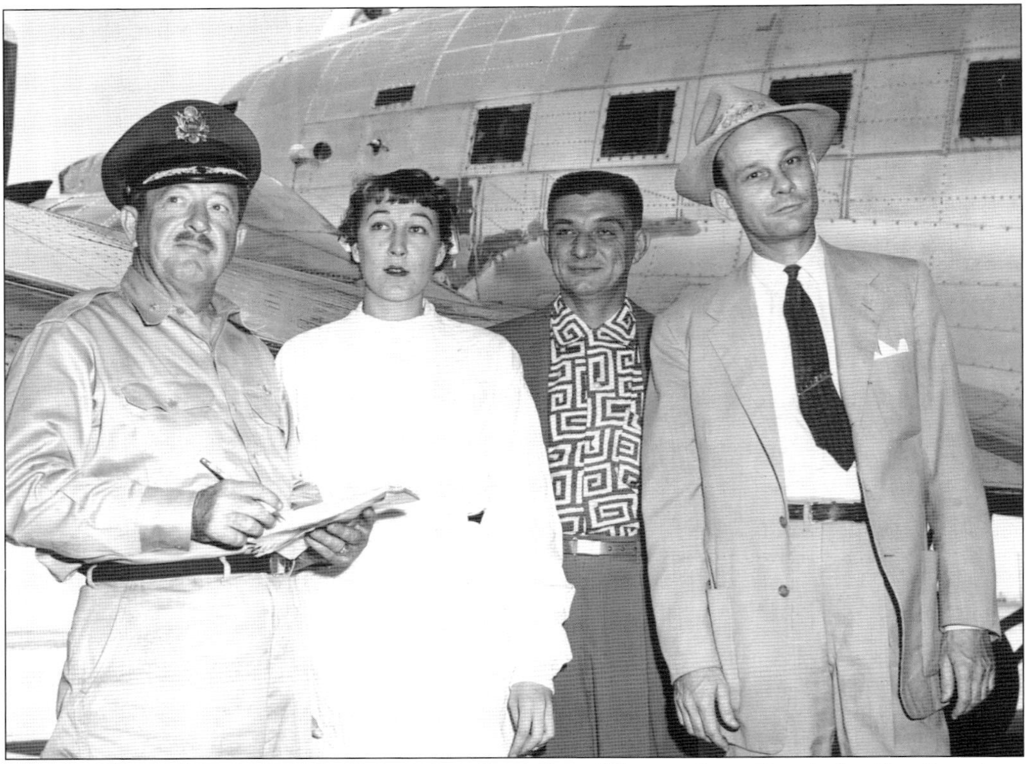

In September 1953, twenty-six patients were flown from Western State Hospital at Fort Supply to Central State Hospital for advanced tuberculosis treatment. The Oklahoma Air National Guard and US Navy coordinated the two flights, which had 13 patients each. Brig. Gen. Maurice Marrs (far left), state air officer, and Maj. Gerald Stevenson (not pictured) piloted the twin-engine C-47 during the two trips. (OHS.)

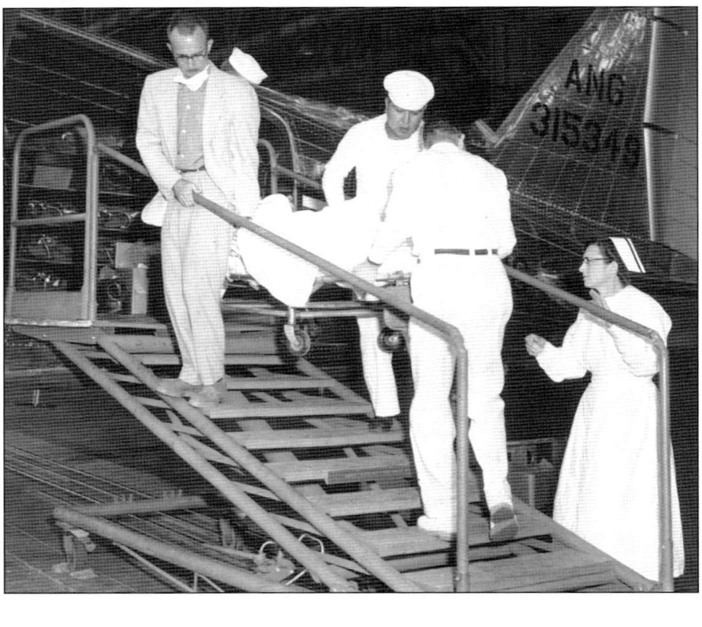

Doctors and nurses helped with the transportation of TB patients, as shown here. Since the mid-1940s, the state health department had traveled the state with portable X-ray machines to scan individuals for tuberculosis. In 1946, there were 6,500 documented cases, although state health officials believed there were twice as many hidden ones. (OHS.)

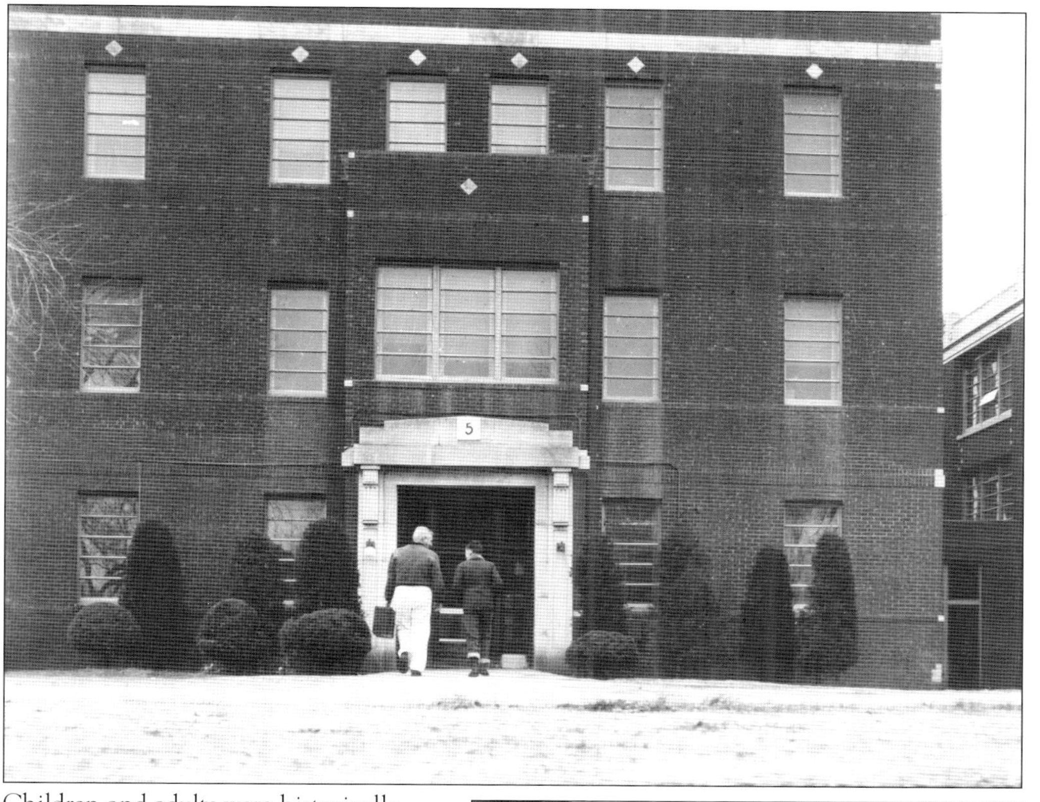

Children and adults were historically housed in the same ward at Central State Hospital. In 1954, the new children's ward (pictured) allowed for 40 children between ages six and fifteen. Housing children in their own ward improved the outlook for their recovery. Administrators also understood that treatments for adults and children were different, and that they had different needs. (OHS.)

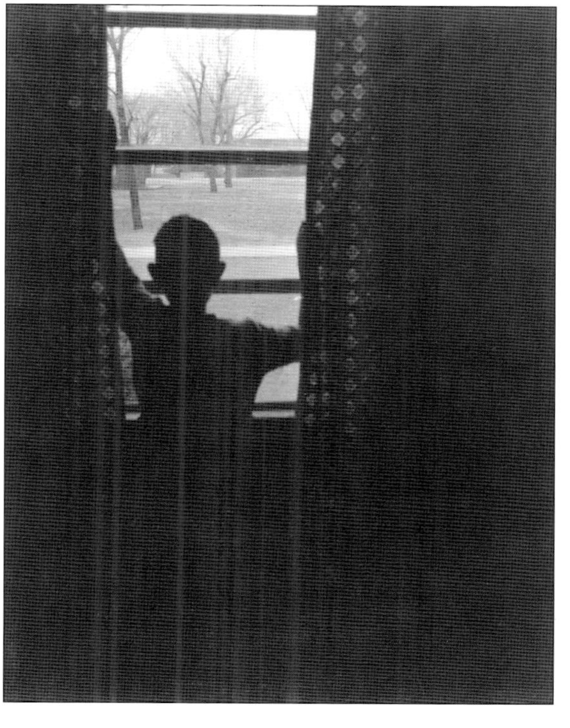

While Dr. Griffin was still superintendent, he believed that some children with mental illness could have been treated by obstetricians, whom he believed needed to be trained in psychiatry so that they could recognize social and psychological problems in children at an early age. The theory that all mental illness was the same in each individual had changed by the 1950s. (OHS.)

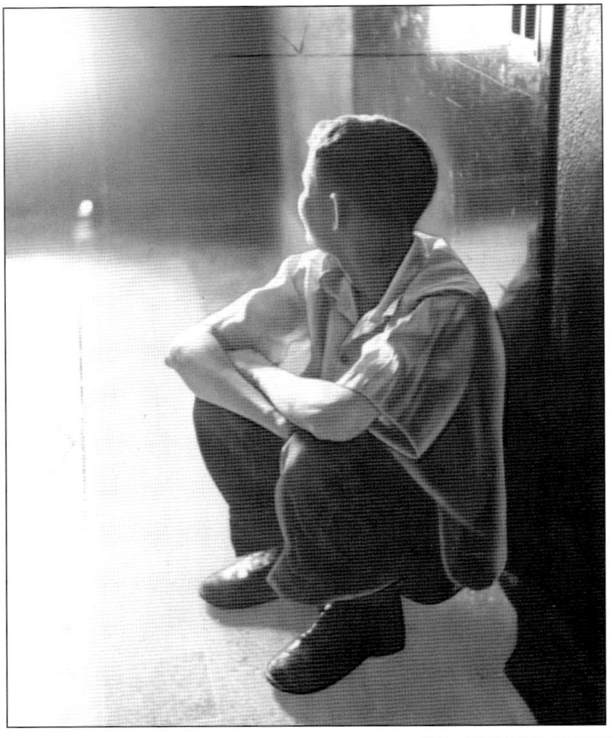

Dr. Hayden Donahue, who was the superintendent in 1961, also believed that not enough attention was given to children with mental illness. He believed there was widespread support for a variety of diseases that strike children, but that most people did not consider mental illness a child's disease and therefore offered very little support or recognition to young people dealing with mental health issues. (OHS.)

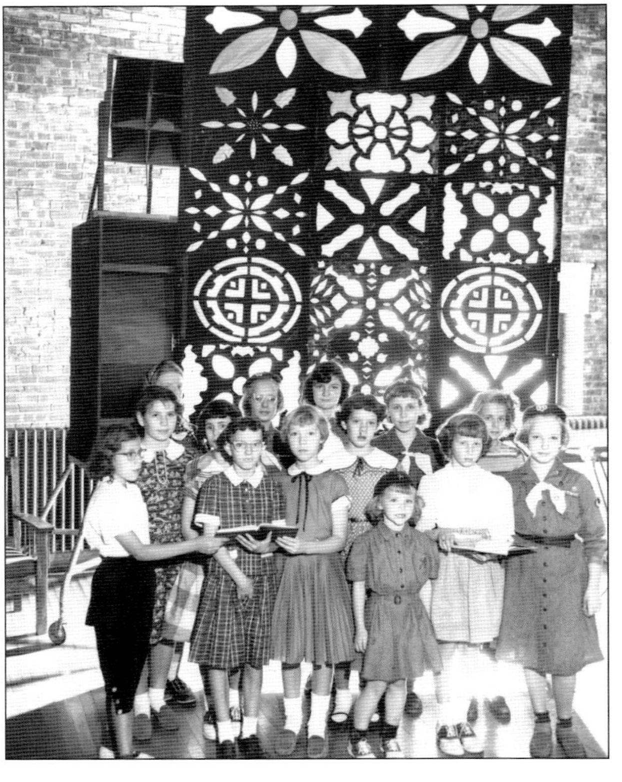

By the late 1950s and 1960s, there was more of a community effort to bring programs to children at Central State Hospital for both entertainment and to uplift their spirits. Groups from the community came to Central State; the Girl Scouts pictured here presented a choir concert that was performed in the American Legion Memorial Chapel. (OHS.)

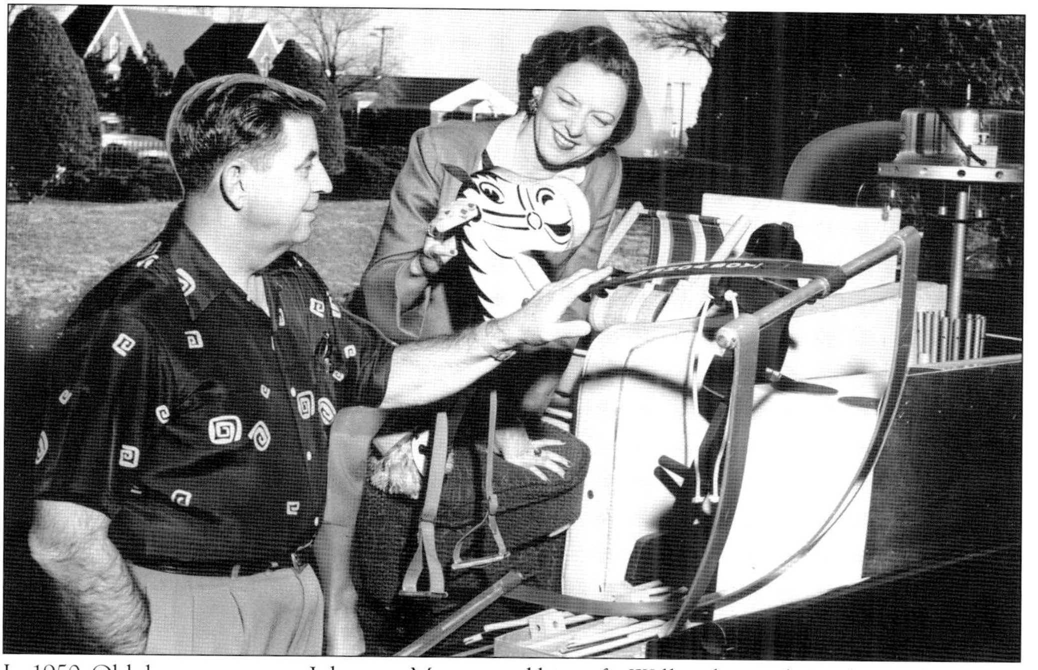

In 1950, Oklahoma governor Johnston Murray and his wife, Willie, donated "Made in Oklahoma" products to the children's ward at Central State Hospital. Murray's sister Jean was a patient at the hospital from 1936 until she died in 1963. Photographs like this one were helpful in Governor Murray's reelection campaign, especially because he was promoting Oklahoma products. (OHS.)

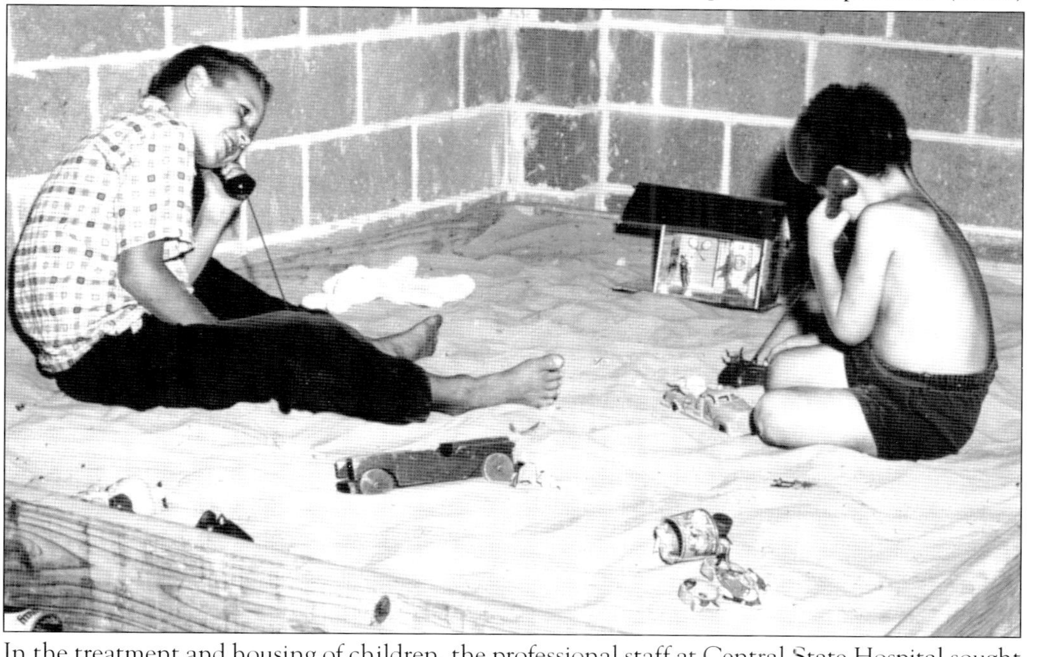

In the treatment and housing of children, the professional staff at Central State Hospital sought to provide an atmosphere that would allow the young people to have an environment conducive to overcoming psychological problems and trauma. Recreational activities were important. (OHS.)

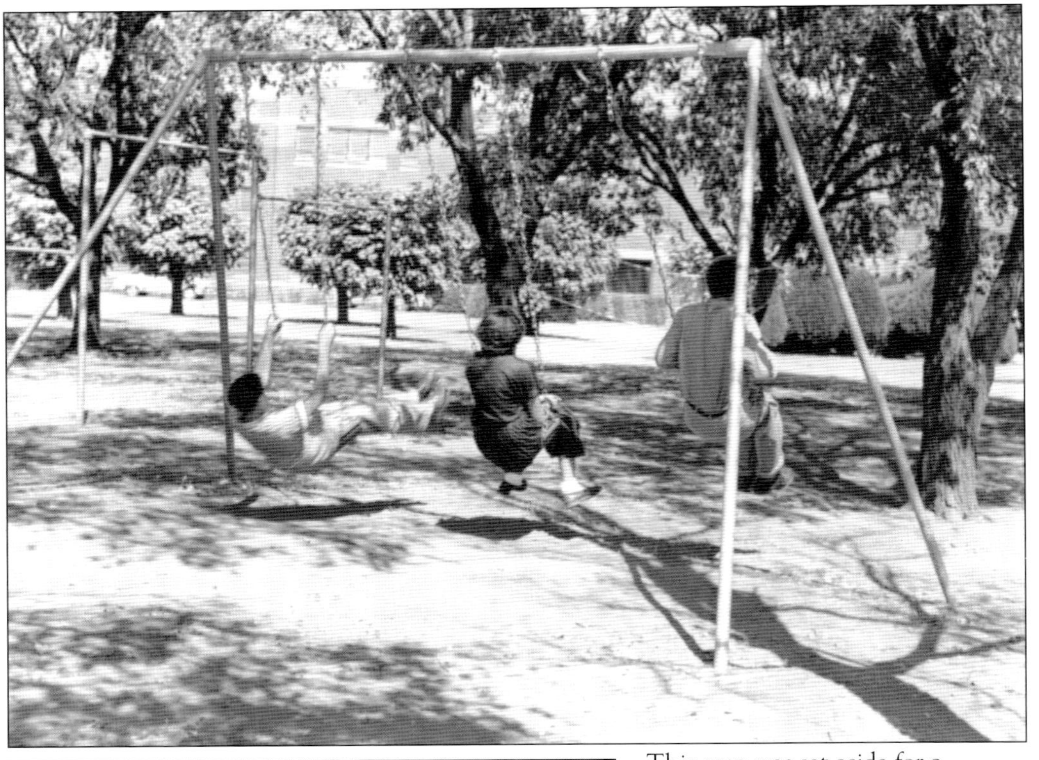

This area was set aside for a playground on Central State Hospital grounds. Although funding was still a problem for administrators and the state legislature, more attention was paid to the children, and more funding was allowed for children's recreation. It was also through the generosity of the Norman community that children at Central State received needed attention. (OHS.)

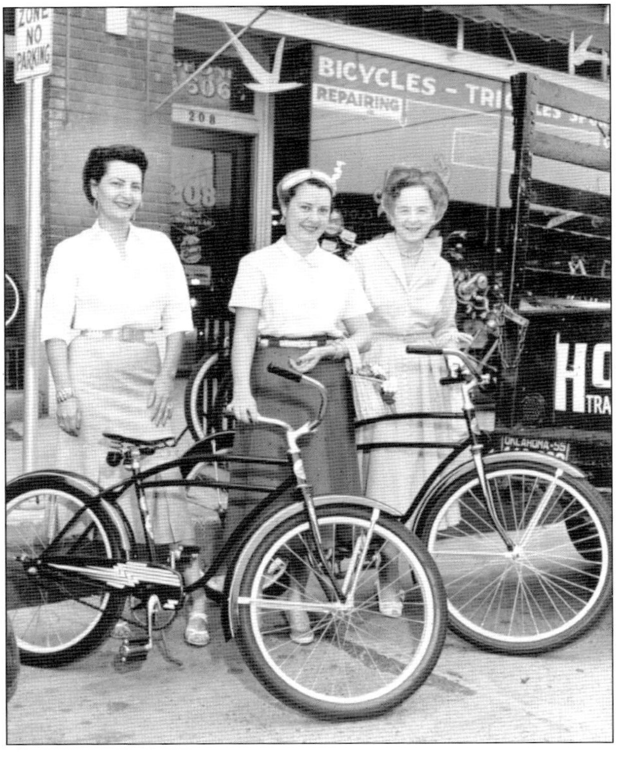

Sororities at the University of Oklahoma found a worthy cause in helping the children at Central State Hospital. The sorority members shown here purchased bicycles for the children. Members of Beta Sigma Phi held a fundraiser to acquire two air conditioners for the wards. Sororities helped needy families at Christmas by donating clothes, magazines, and sundry gifts to patients. (OHS.)

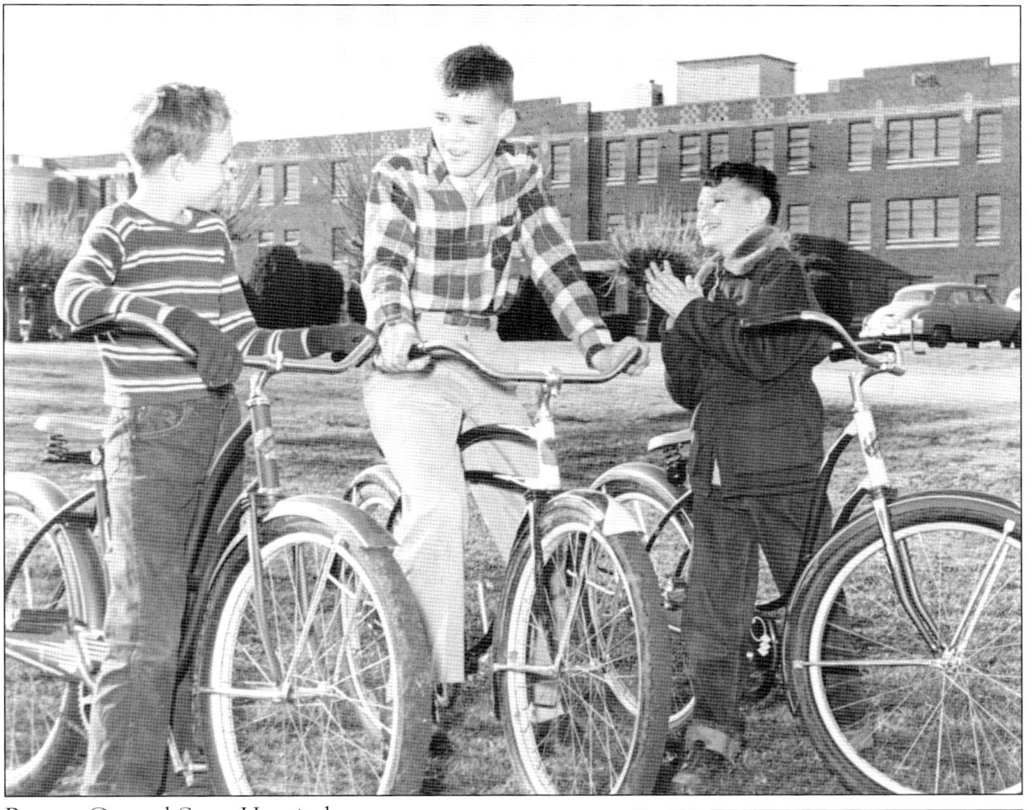

Boys at Central State Hospital enjoyed riding the bicycles provided by members of the University of Oklahoma sororities. The Beta Eta chapter organized a number of charitable drives. With the proceeds from these drives, they purchased a piano for the adult ward, as well as furniture for the children's reception room and necessary items for the children's ward. (OHS.)

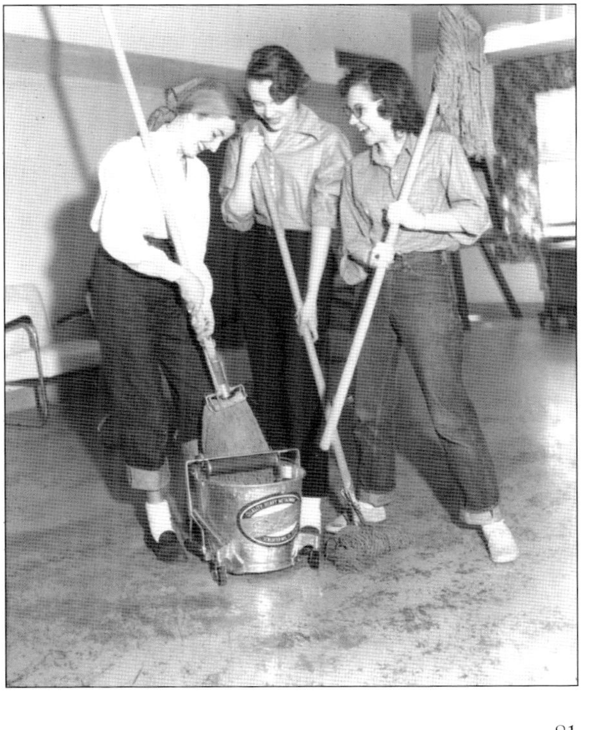

In 1955, these sorority pledges from the University of Oklahoma helped clean wards as part of their obligation and commitment to service. Many charitable organizations raised funds to provide things for children at the hospital, including modeling clay, books, model airplanes, toys, earmuffs, footballs, basketballs, and an assortment of items suitable for boys or girls. (OHS.)

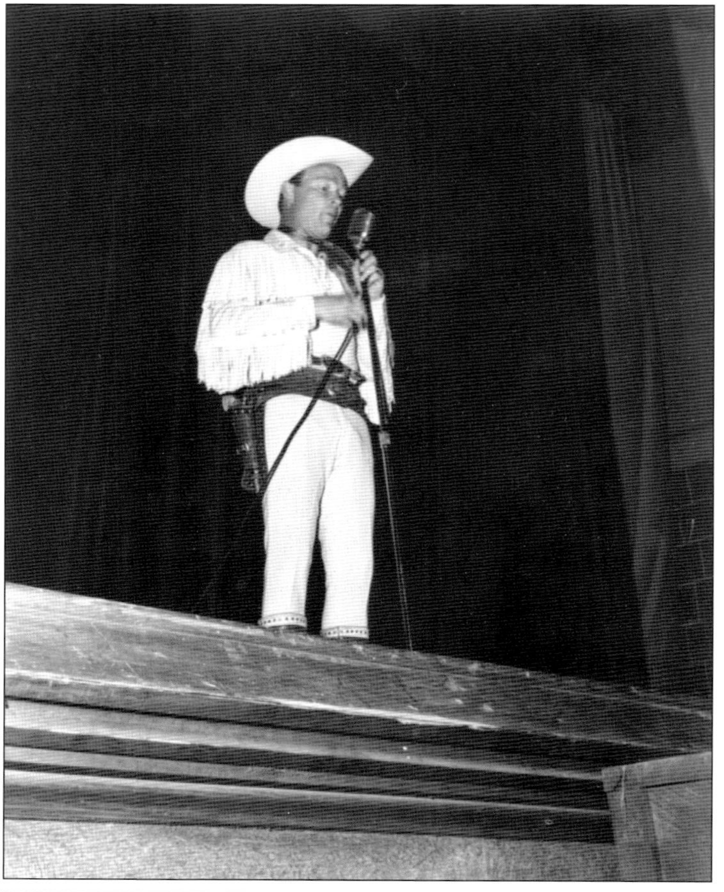

Popular actor Roy Rogers visited Central State Hospital in May 1954. He was in Oklahoma to attend a ground-breaking ceremony for a new building for children who had speech and hearing defects. The fundraisers asked children to donate 10¢ to enter a contest to name the new building. Eleven winners received a variety of gifts, including a Shetland pony, $100, Nellybelle Jeeps, and new cowboy outfits. (OHS.)

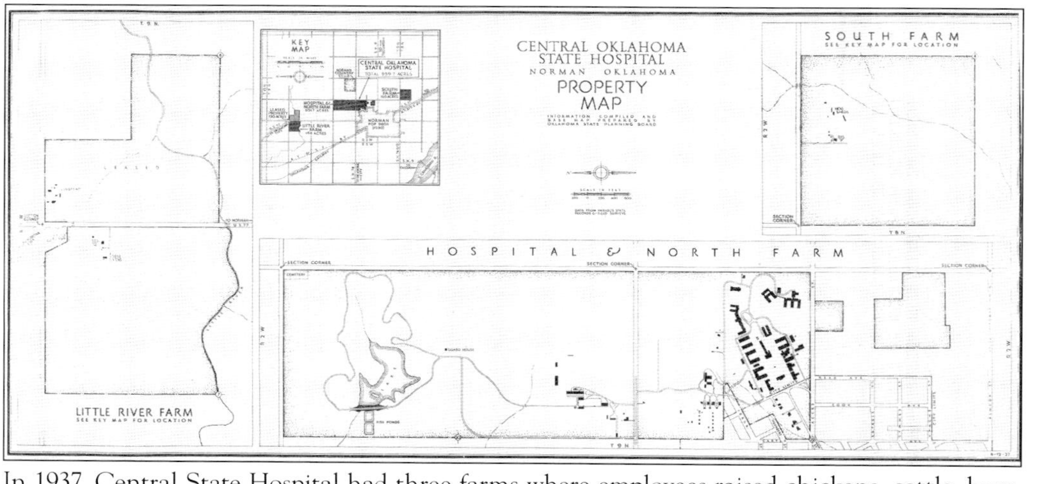

In 1937, Central State Hospital had three farms where employees raised chickens, cattle, hogs, and goats. To the north of the main hospital, near the present-day intersection of Robinson Street and Southeast Twelfth Avenue, was a 320-acre farm; at US 77 and Franklin Road, there was a 180-acre farm; and at Lindsey Street and Porter Avenue, there was a 150-acre farm called South Farm. These farms supplied the hospital with meat and vegetables. (OHC.)

As early as 1919, Central State Hospital, under the supervision of Dr. Griffin, was recognized for breeding quality cattle and cows. An advertisement in the *Duncan Weekly Eagle* announced the sale of "Choice Calves to 2-year-old, including son of Lady Hermel." Lady Hermel was evidently prized for her yearly production of 11,040 pounds of milk and 678 pounds of butter. (OHS.)

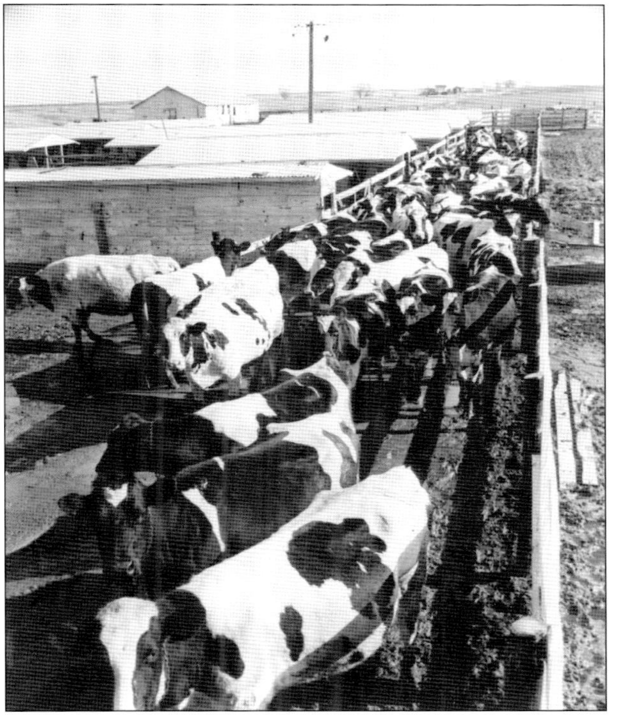

The 320-acre farm at Robinson Street and Southeast Twelfth Avenue, north of Central State Hospital, was primarily a dairy farm and locally known as the Jersey Farm. The farm housed 250 cows that supplied 800 to 850 gallons of milk per year. Twenty-five patients worked at the facility. Livestock from the farm was shown in county and state fairs and usually won first place. (OHS.)

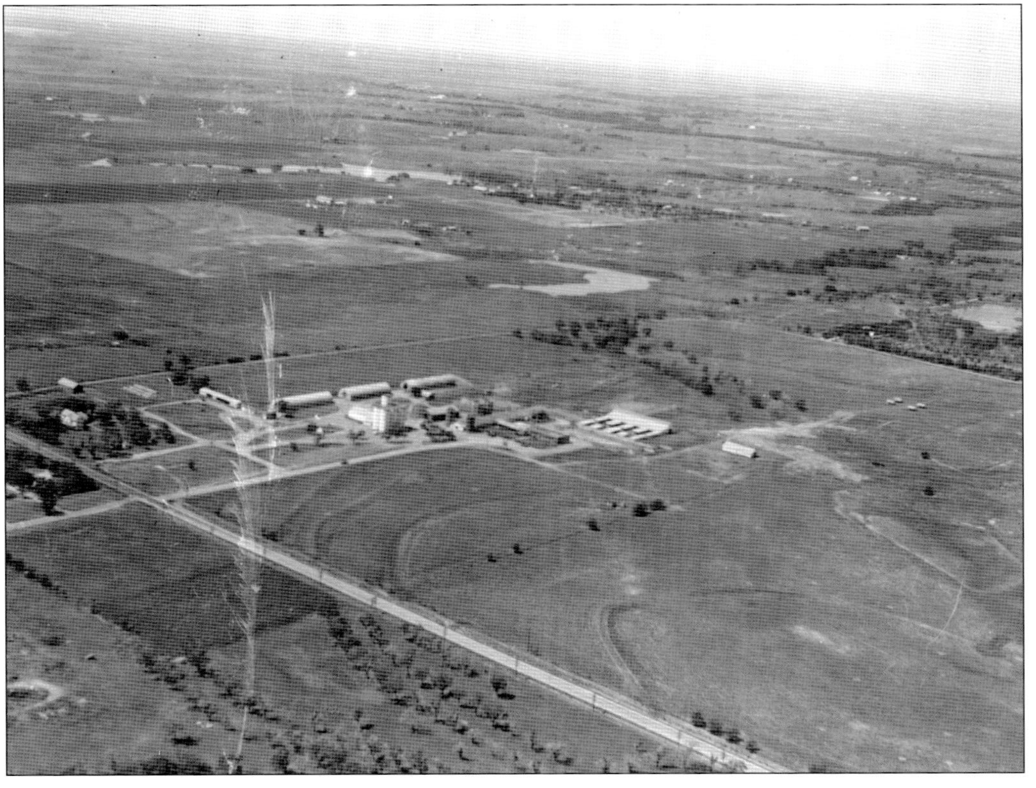

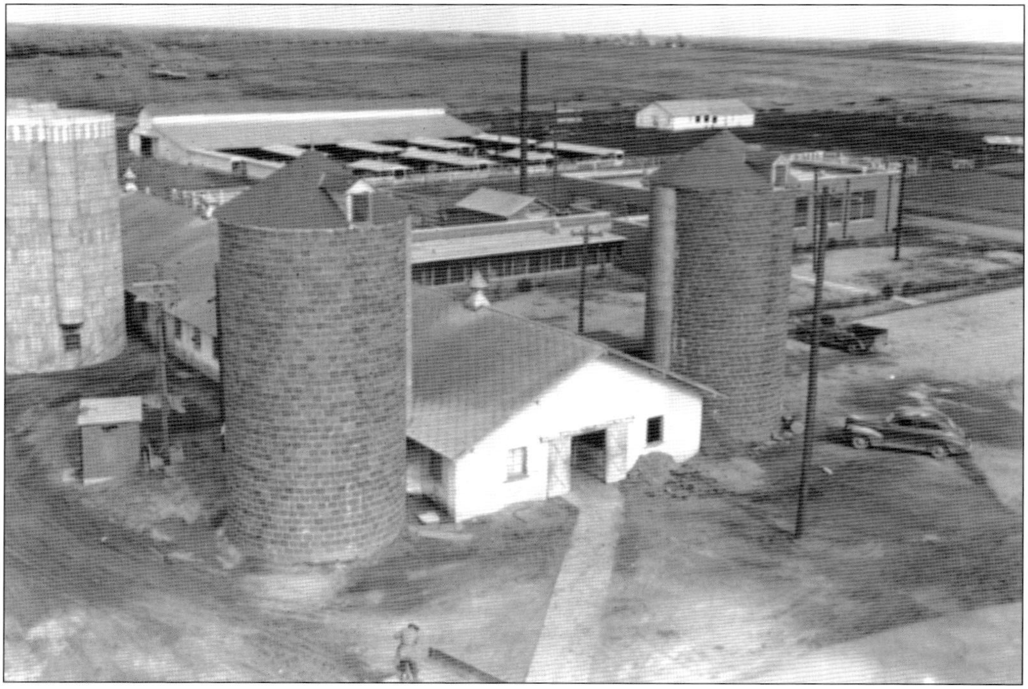

The administration and employees at Central State Hospital were proud of their farms and farm production, which helped to feed patients at the hospital. The quality of the farms was judged by the output from the dairy cows. In 1929, Central State cows produced a record amount of butterfat (an average of 39.1 pounds) from eight Jersey cows and eleven Holsteins. (OHS.)

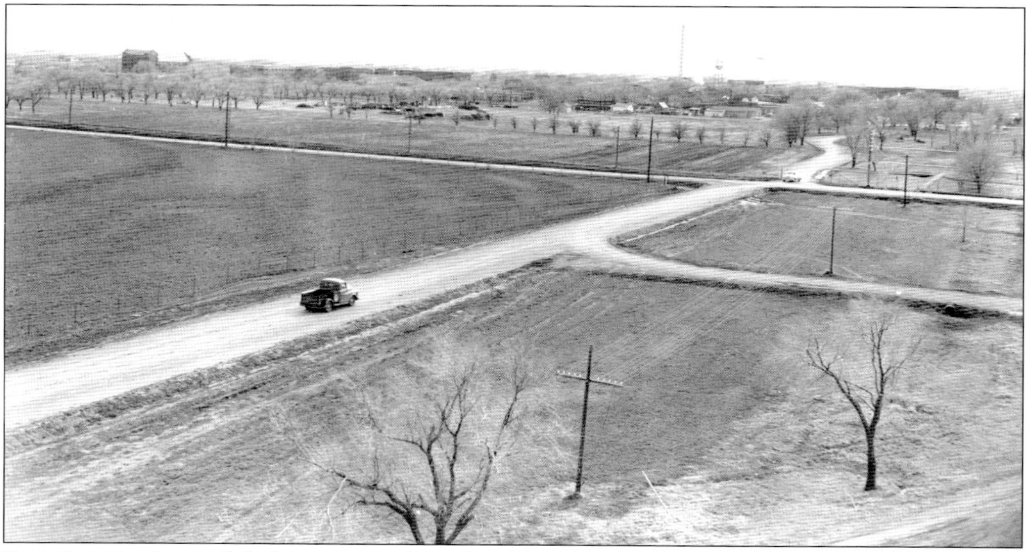

Each farm had a qualified superintendent. In 1952, Von H. Long was named supervisor of farm operations at Central State Hospital. Previously, he was the district supervisor of the veterans' agricultural program. Long obtained a master's degree in agriculture from Oklahoma State University. At Central State, he was in charge of 1,300 acres of hospital land and 1,800 acres of leased land. (OHS.)

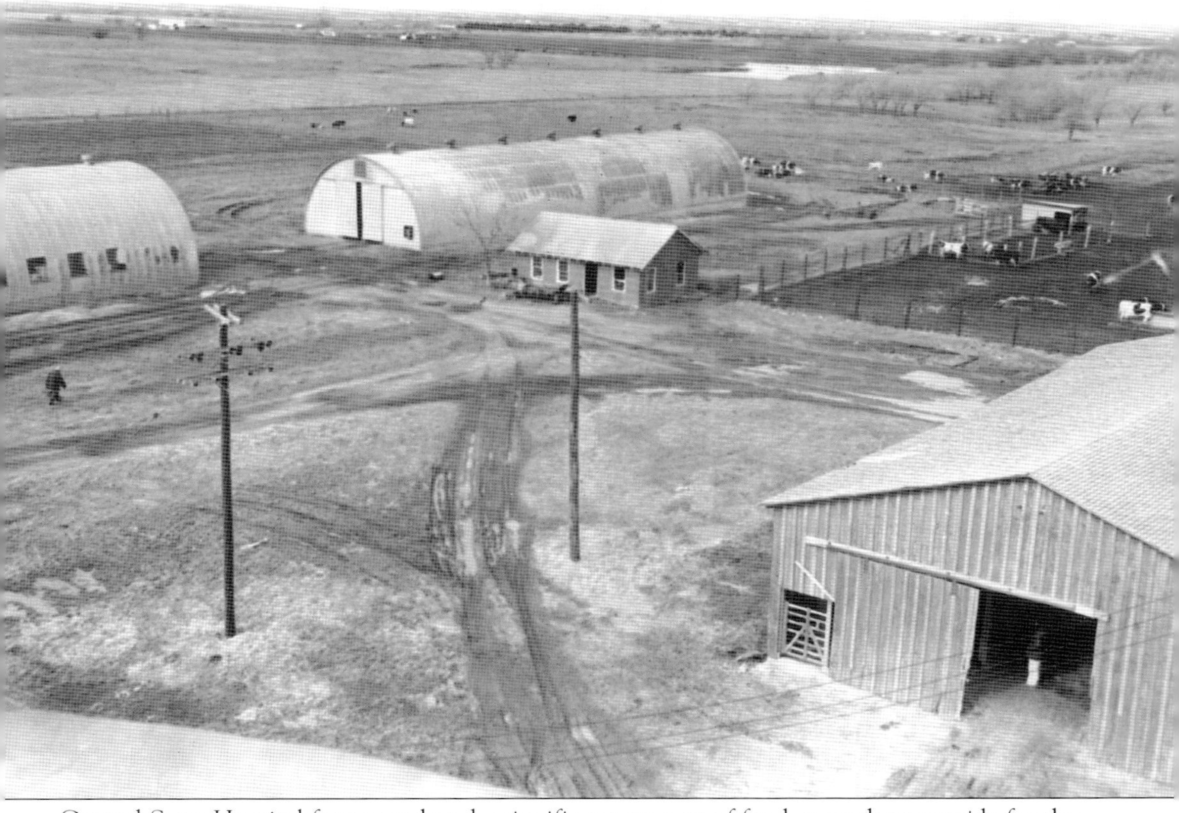

Central State Hospital farms produced a significant amount of food, enough to provide for the needs of 3,000 patients depending on the years of production. In 1930, the production of milk and butter over an 11-month period totaled $53,077, with the surplus sold to the public. By the 1940s, there were 78 patients from Central State working on the farm. They grew Irish and sweet potatoes, roasting ear corn, black-eyed peas, alfalfa hay, corn, oats, sweet clover, seed straw, hay, and cotton. In 1941, farm production provided 25 percent of the cost of food. It was reported, however, that the patients' diets were lacking in nutritional value. For example, a typical diet was bread, milk, fresh tomatoes, pumpkin, pinto beans, peanut butter, and peaches. On some days, the offering was bread, milk, peaches, bologna, and beet pickles. (OHS.)

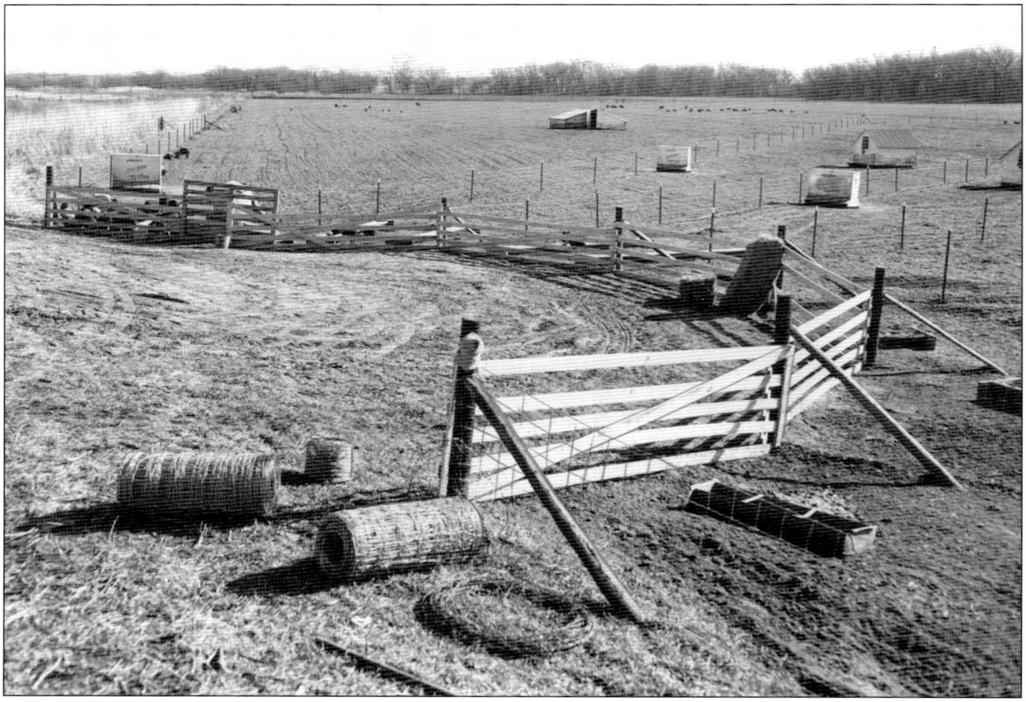

The agricultural land owned by Central State Hospital near present-day Hollywood Corners at North Porter Avenue and Franklin Road was productive if there was not too much rain. Charles Hogan, one of the managers of Central State farmlands, complained to the city on a regular basis about the flooding every time there was significant rain. (OHS.)

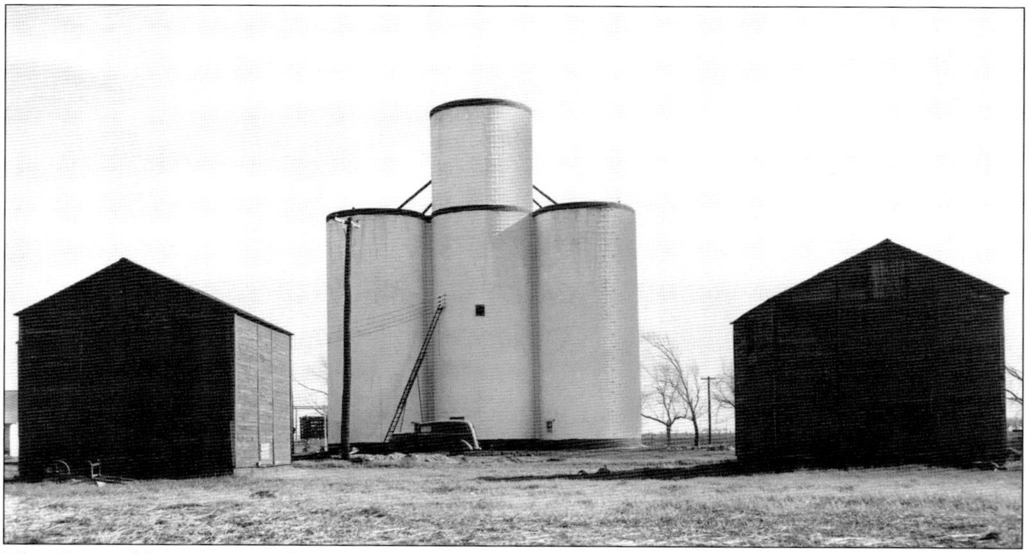

The Central State Hospital farm at Robinson Street and Southeast Twelfth Avenue was known for prize hogs that were raised on the farm and known as Hampshire Porkers. Today, the silos pictured here stand as the only testament to the extremely productive farming operation at Central State, one of the most successful in Cleveland County. (OHS.)

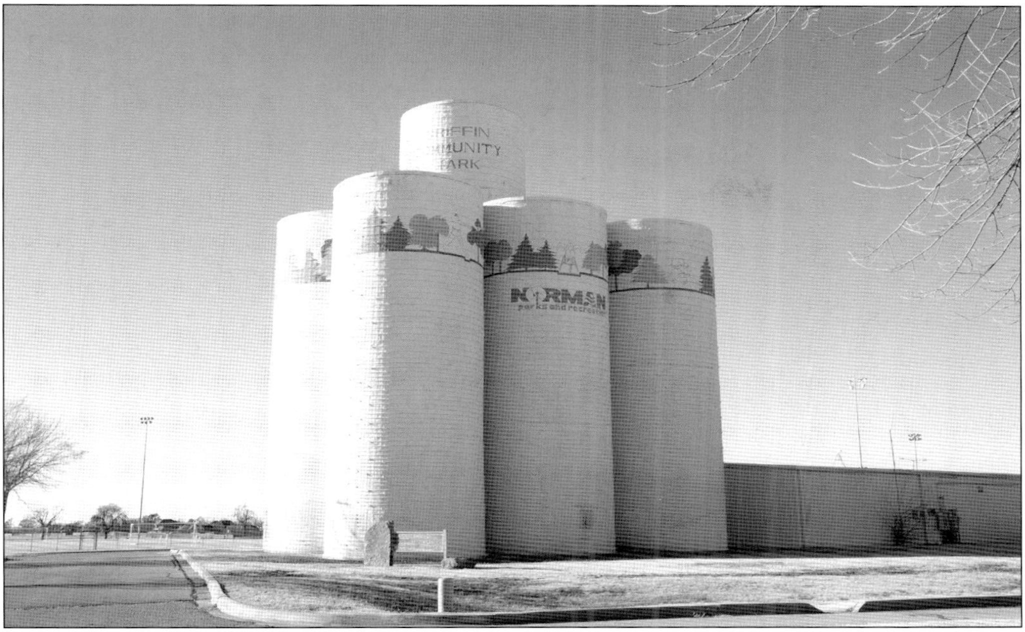

The farm at Robinson Street and Southeast Twelfth Avenue was bought by the City of Norman for use by Norman's parks and recreation department. What was once a farm is now divided into soccer and baseball fields. All that remains of the old farm are the silos, which became a historic landmark. (CCHS.)

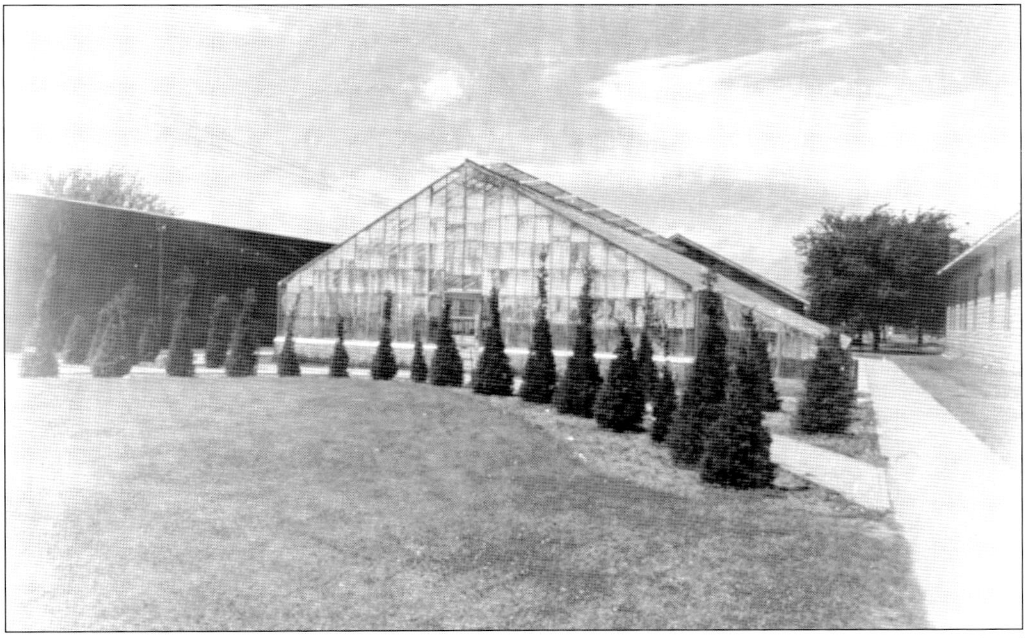

Besides meat and dairy products, Central State Hospital grew vegetables on the hospital's farmland and had a small orchard on the main grounds just south of the hospital buildings. This greenhouse was one of the agricultural features of the hospital. All Central State farm output was produced for the benefit of the patients. (CCHS.)

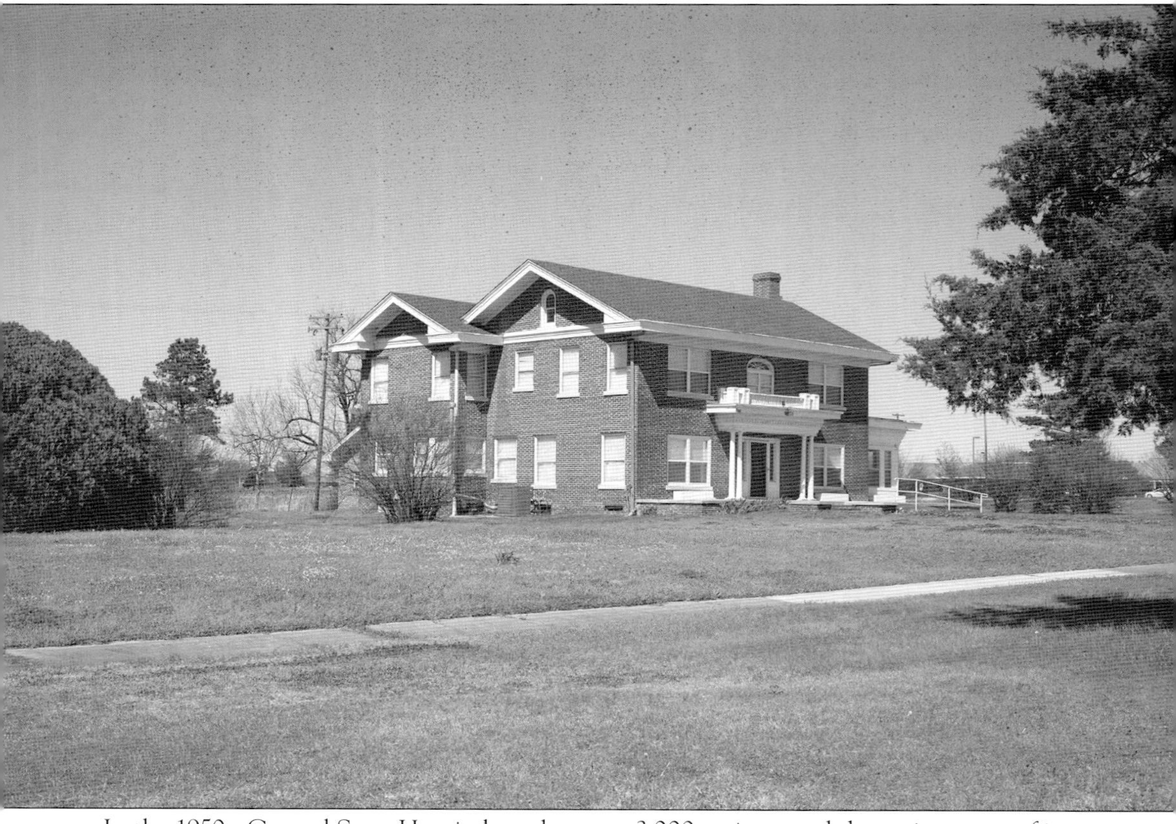

In the 1950s, Central State Hospital was home to 3,000 patients and the main source of income for many who worked at the hospital: attendants, doctors, nurses, and other staff members. The hospital was the home of the superintendents who were in charge of the facility over the years. This is the superintendent's residence, which was on the north side of the tree-lined main entrance to the hospital grounds. (CCHS.)

Five

More Changes 1950s

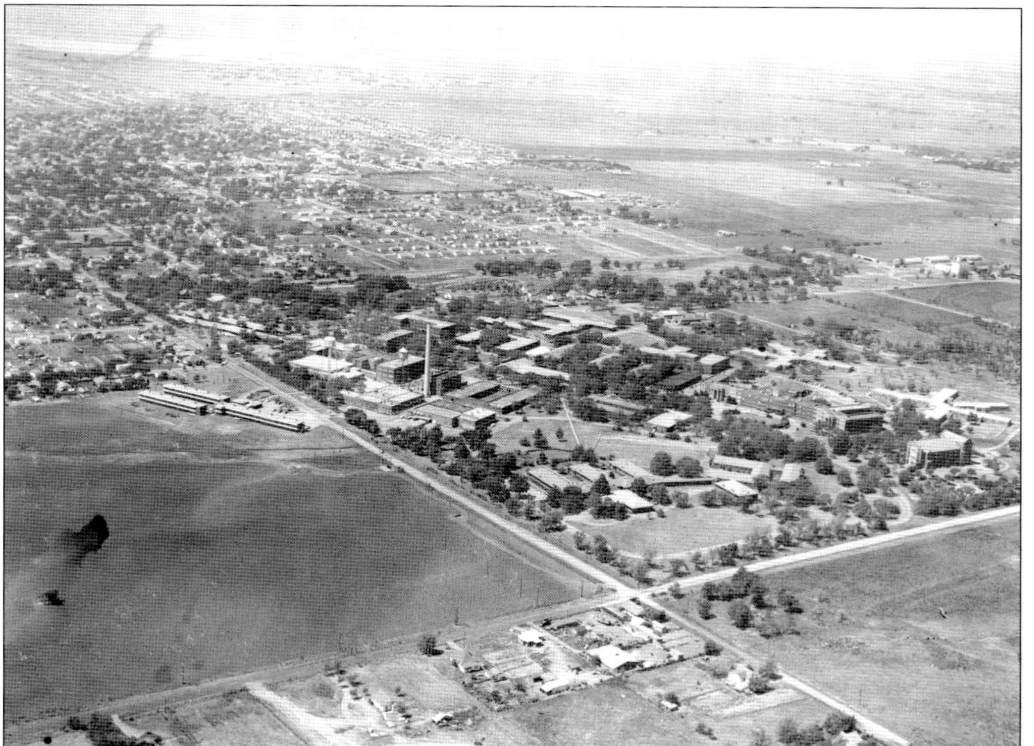

Dr. David Griffin was employed at Central State Hospital for 51 years. He passed away in 1953, three years after his retirement from the hospital. Some state legislators sought to rename the hospital in honor of Griffin after he retired in 1950; there was opposition to the name change until after Griffin's death. Legislators agreed to change the name of the institution to Central State Griffin Memorial Hospital in 1958. (OHS.)

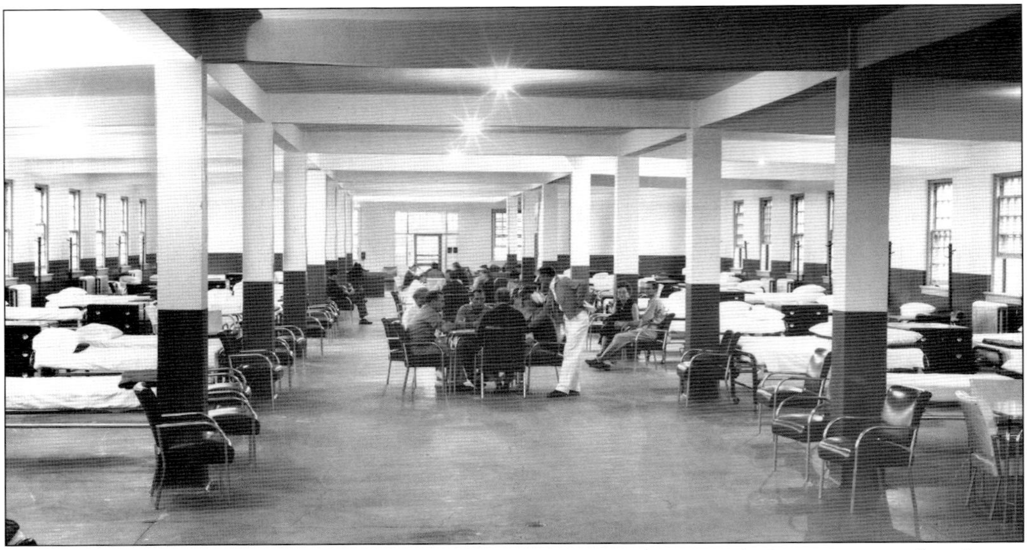

Two things brought change for patients at Griffin Memorial Hospital. One was state legislative approval of new nursing standards, which included required courses in psychiatric care. By 1958, Griffin Memorial offered courses in mental health that fulfilled state requirements. Becoming a teaching hospital brought needed professional staff (shown here in a meeting) who helped to improve patient care. (OHS.)

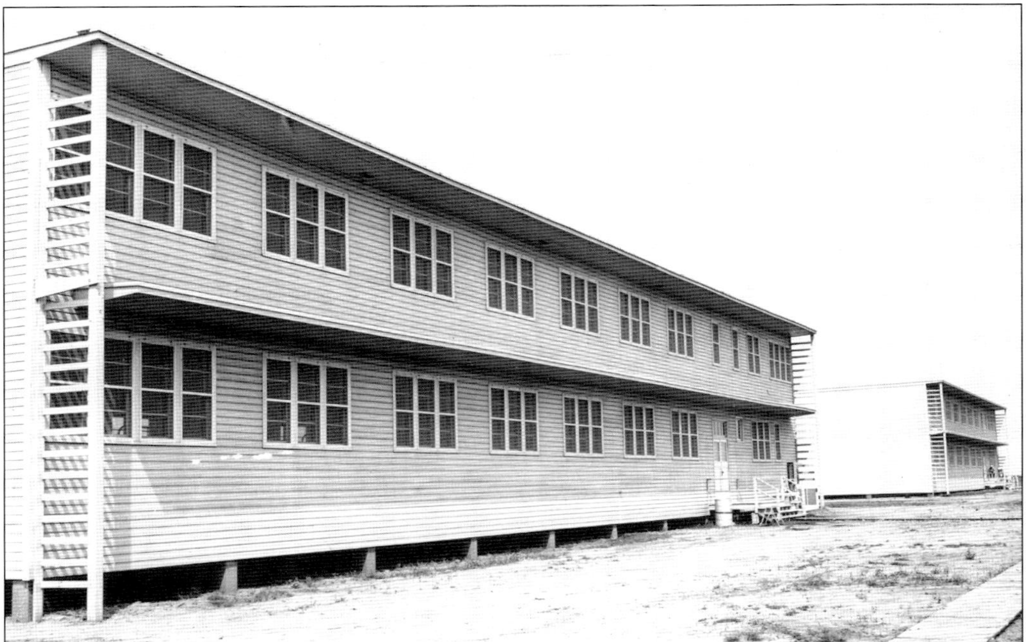

Until official housing was completed, the University of Oklahoma offered dorm space for nursing students in barracks at the former World War II Naval Air Technical Training Center or South Base. The university owned the base land and buildings. South Base was located just southeast of the University of Oklahoma campus. (OHS.)

In 1950, the Oklahoma legislature allocated $3,256,725 for the construction of two buildings at Griffin Memorial Hospital. The new ward building that housed 400 patients was at the northeast edge of the property. The other building (pictured) was for nurses and employees. This building was constructed on the south side of East Main Street. (OHS.)

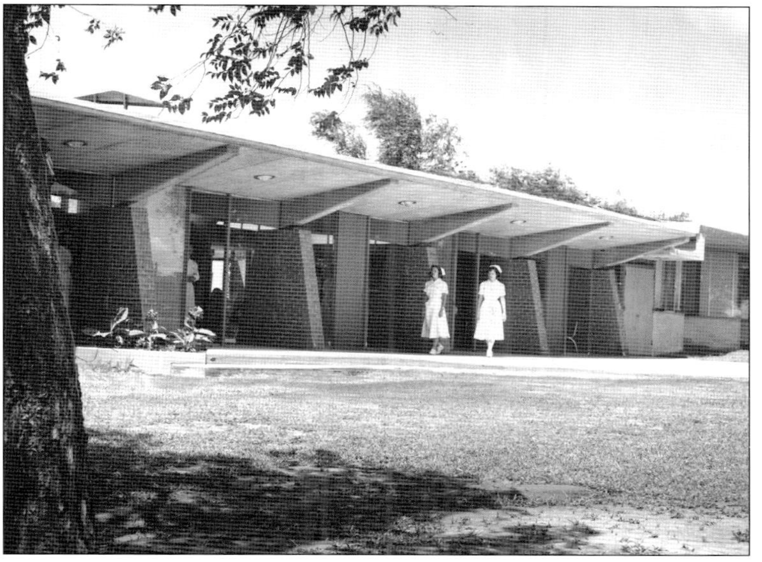

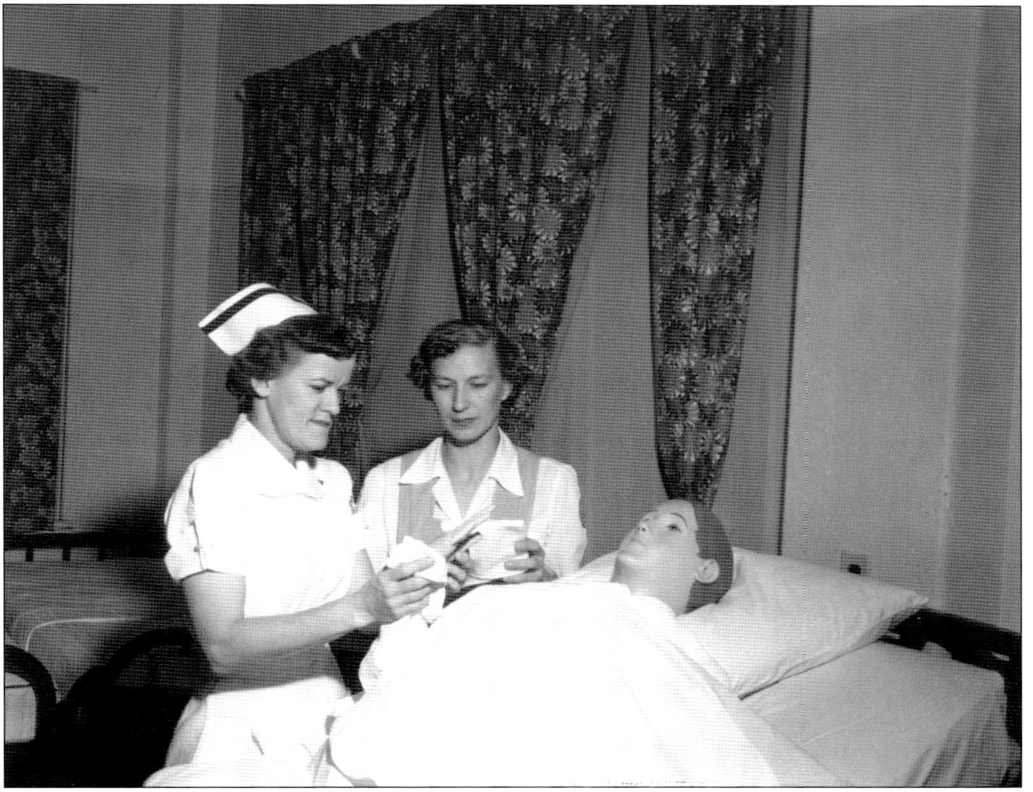

In 1950, a new state law that required the completion of a three-month nursing program in psychiatric training before graduation resulted in 58 student nurses becoming the first class at Griffin Memorial. Previously, student nurses had to leave the state to receive psychiatric training. At Griffin, students received training in psychiatry, social service, neurology, occupational therapy, and special therapies. (OHS.)

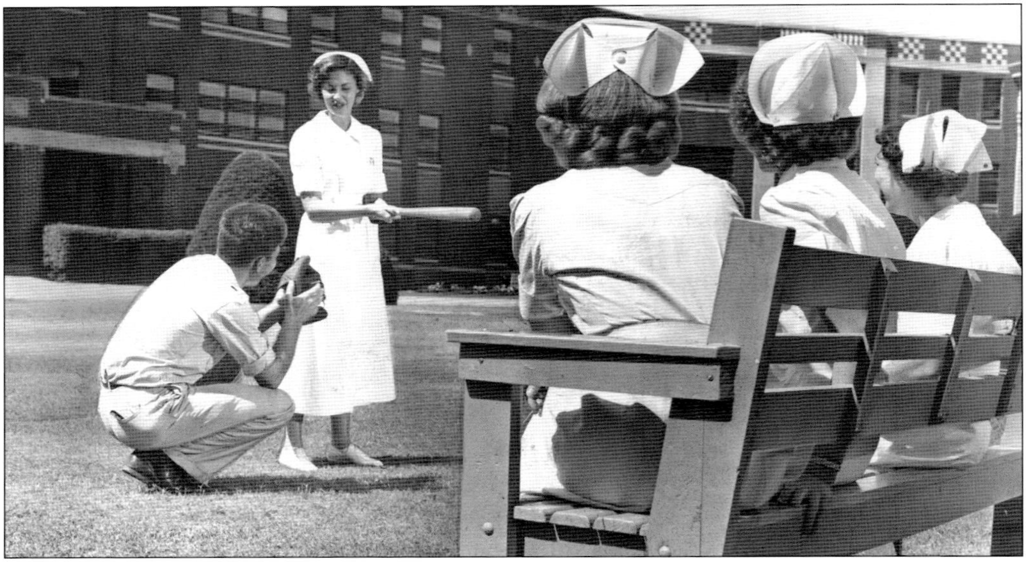

Nurses were also trained in a variety of occupational and recreational therapies. Each student spent two weeks working in the occupational therapy ward. The nurses helped patients to knit, sew, paint, and crochet; patients also participated in rug-making and leatherworking. The students also played baseball, card games, and drop-the-handkerchief, as well as helping young girls to dress their dolls. (OHS.)

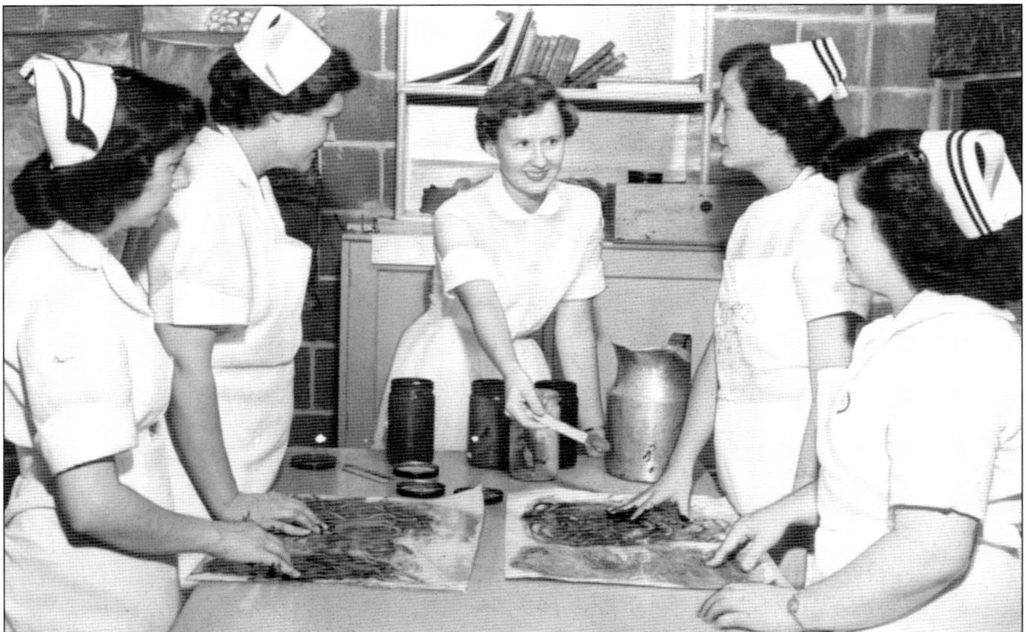

Working with different arts and crafts became an important part of a patient's well-being. Nurses who were trained in occupational and recreational therapy sought to bring out the creative parts of a patient's personality. Helping patients to develop their own creativity became part of a nurse's training. The popular belief was that any attention given to the patient's creativity helped nudge them toward strong mental health. (OHS.)

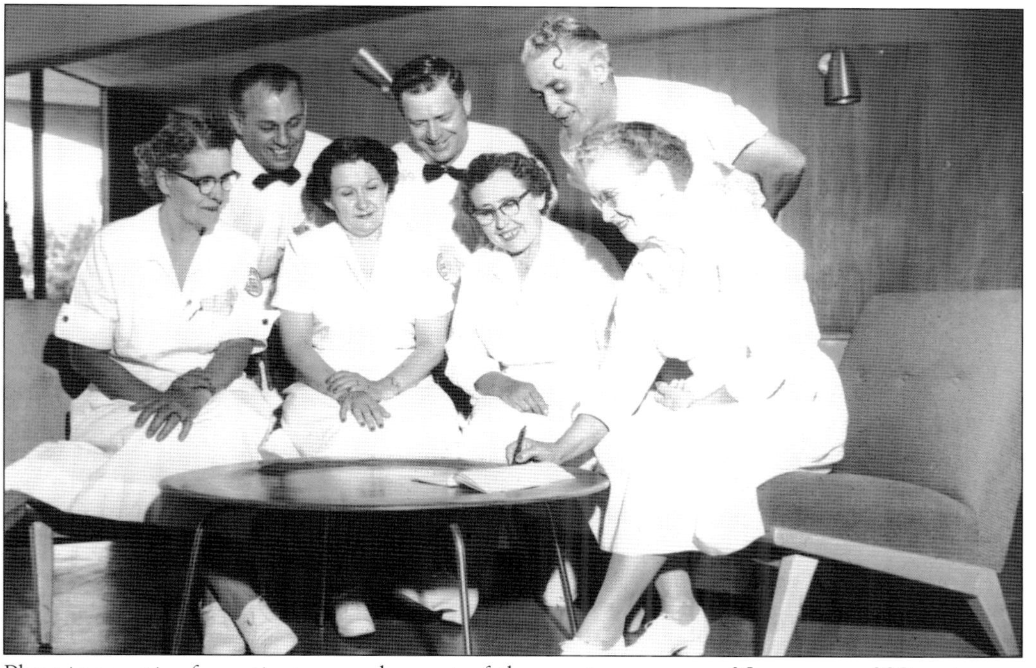

Planning parties for patients was also part of the nursing program. Nurses gave 300 patients a Valentine's Day party at the American Legion Memorial Chapel. In 1953, the nurses asked patients to present musical programs and skits. The afternoon program was made up of a hillbilly band, a dancing-doll skit, tap-dancing, and a comedy act. After refreshments, nurses and patients danced to music provided by the hospital orchestra. (OHS.)

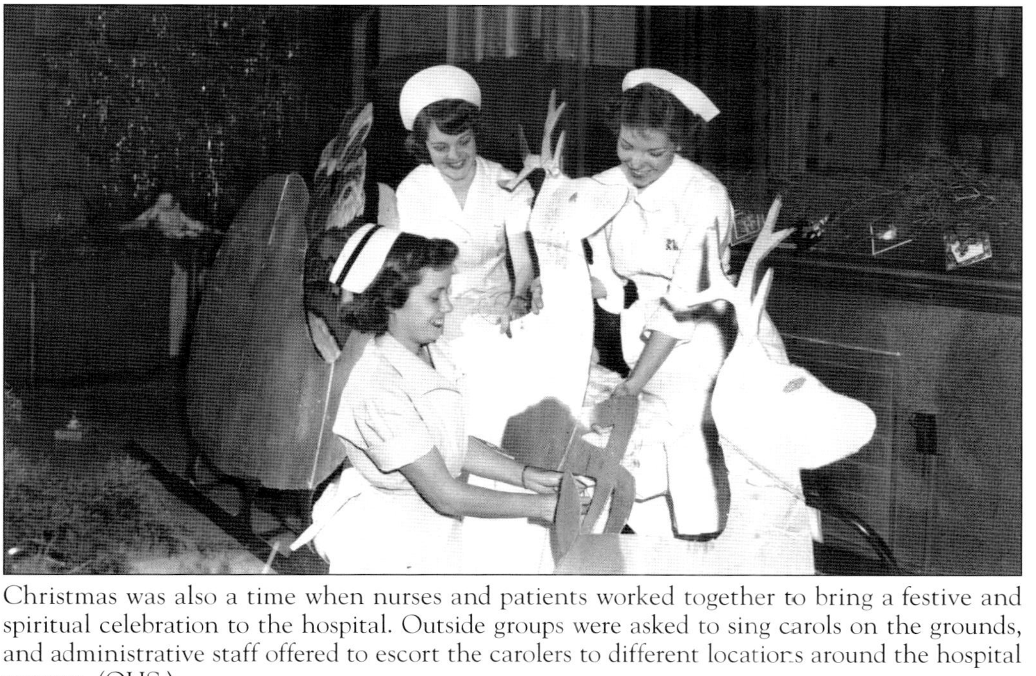

Christmas was also a time when nurses and patients worked together to bring a festive and spiritual celebration to the hospital. Outside groups were asked to sing carols on the grounds, and administrative staff offered to escort the carolers to different locations around the hospital campus. (OHS.)

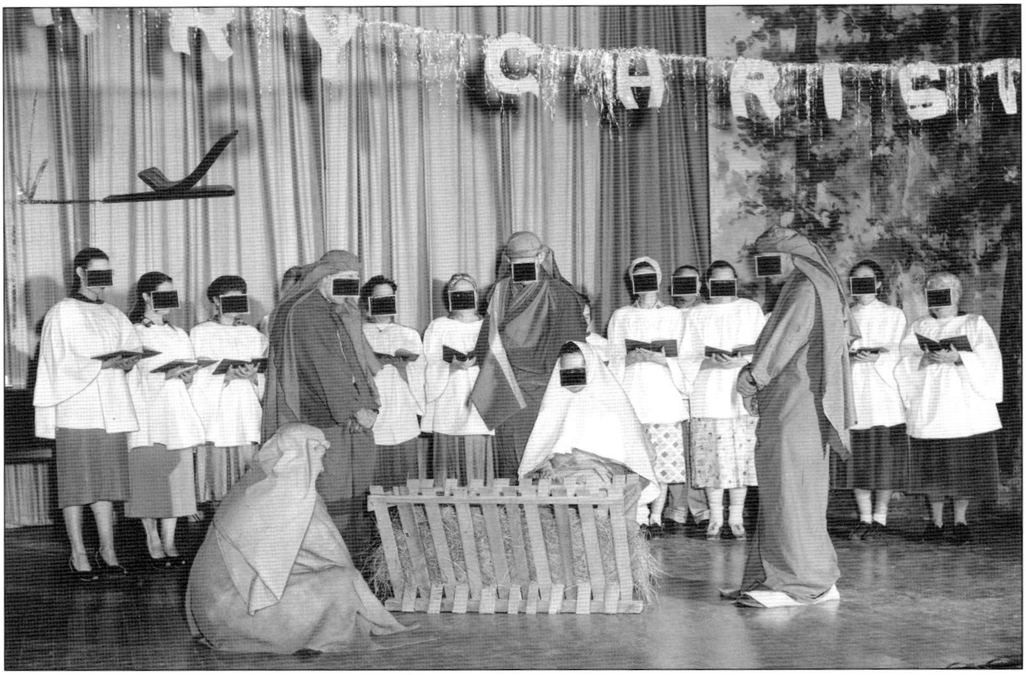

Nurses helped the patients to present Christmas programs and helped them decorate their wards. Along with the caroling, patients had the opportunity to visit Santa. Volunteers organized the donation of gifts for each of the 3,000 patients at the hospital. The list of suitable gifts included socks, cigarettes, candy, stationery, combs, scarves, bobby pins, house shoes, and perfumed soap. The choir included Griffin Memorial patients. (OHS.)

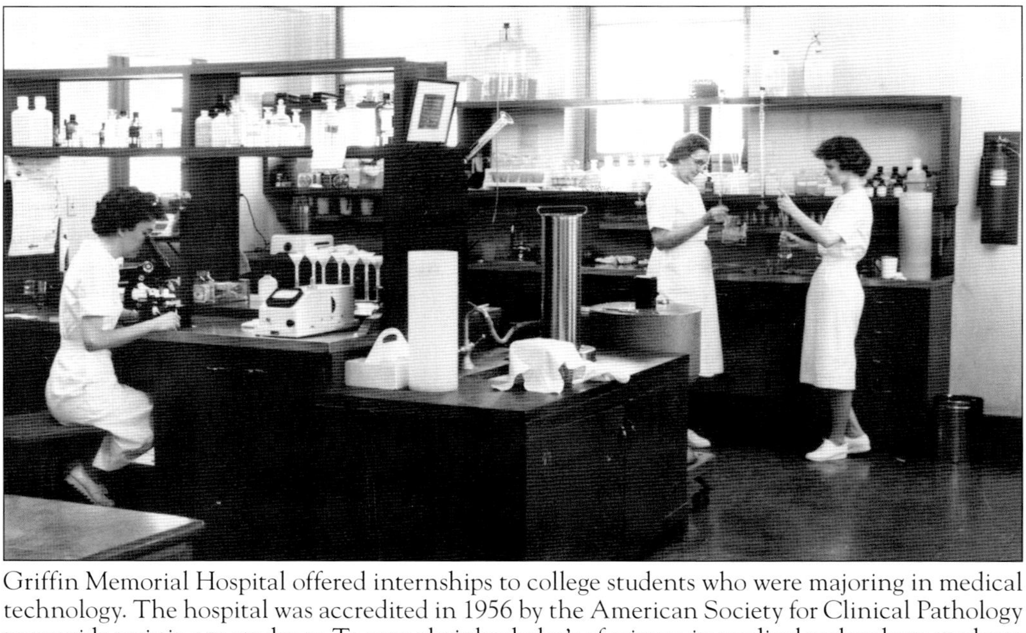

Griffin Memorial Hospital offered internships to college students who were majoring in medical technology. The hospital was accredited in 1956 by the American Society for Clinical Pathology to provide training to students. To earn their bachelor's of science in medical technology, students worked for a year at the hospital from 8:00 a.m. to 5:00 p.m., five days per week. (OHS.)

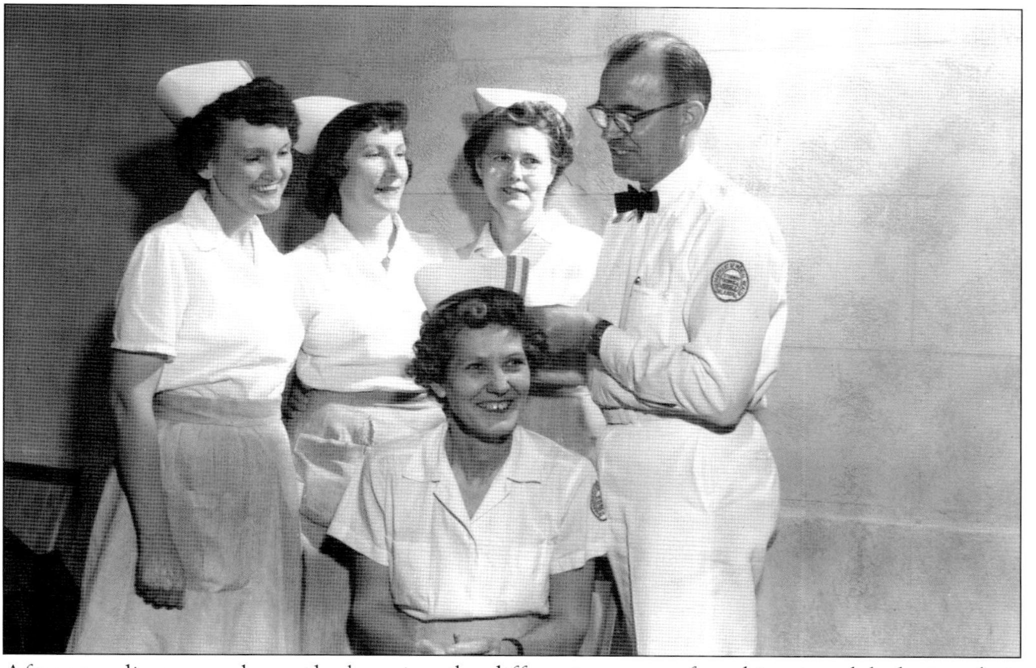

After spending several months learning the different aspects of working in a lab during their coursework and working in the wards with patients using their knowledge of occupational and physical therapy, each trainee graduated and left Griffin Memorial Hospital. A new class of nurse trainees then started the training courses. (OHS.)

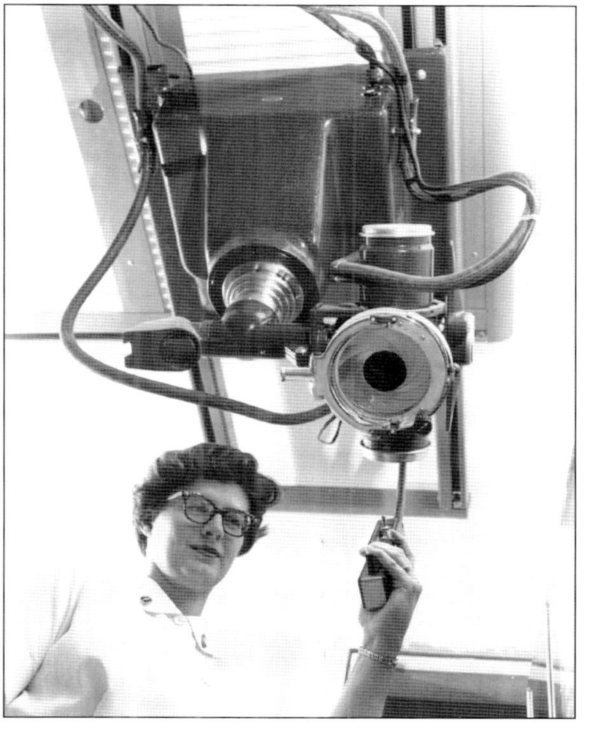

In 1955, Griffin Memorial Hospital was keeping up with new medical trends in Oklahoma hospitals. Acquiring an X-ray machine and establishing a department of radiology was one such trend. Portable X-ray machines were in wide use across the state as a way to diagnose tuberculosis in the general population. At Griffin, the X-ray machine served in the treatment of TB and in diagnosing injuries. Some nurses trained in radiology. (OHS.)

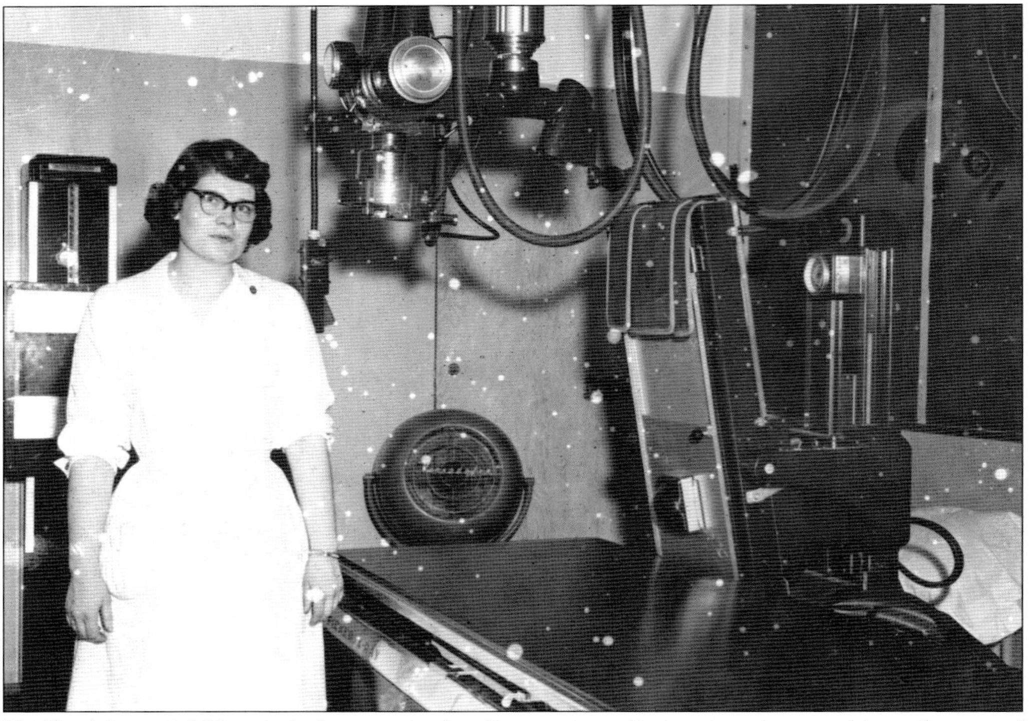

Griffin Memorial Hospital also acquired a diagnostic radiation imaging machine, the use of which involved an application of contrast agents that could be used to provide a better image and contrast for organ visualization. This picture from a *Daily Oklahoman* article shows a radiological technician standing beside Griffin Memorial's X-ray and imaging equipment. (OHS.)

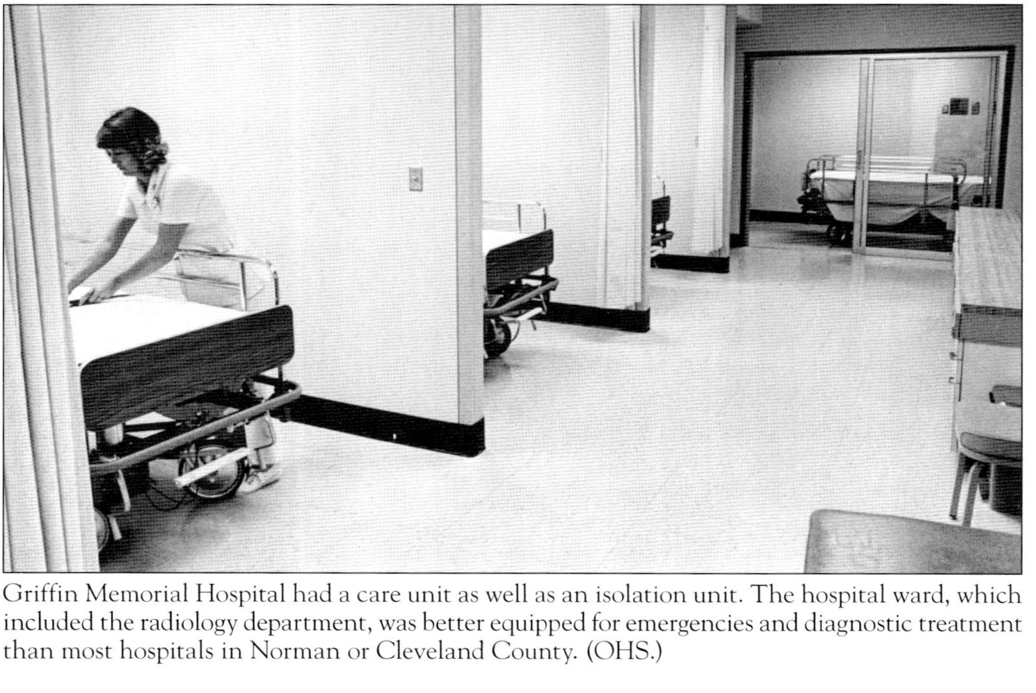

Griffin Memorial Hospital had a care unit as well as an isolation unit. The hospital ward, which included the radiology department, was better equipped for emergencies and diagnostic treatment than most hospitals in Norman or Cleveland County. (OHS.)

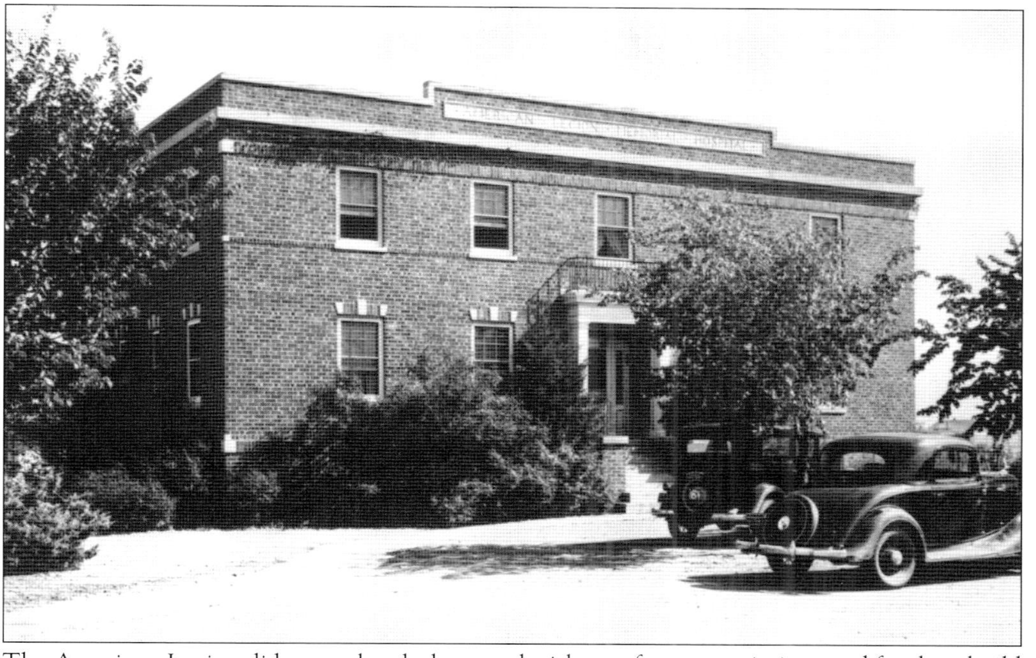

The American Legion did not only ask the state legislature for appropriations and funds to build a veterans' hospital and wards at Central State Hospital. In 1925, the Legion acquired funds to build Norman's first hospital at Johnson and North Ponca Streets. The hospital was erected in honor of those who fought in the First World War. With additions, this became Norman Regional Hospital. (CCHS.)

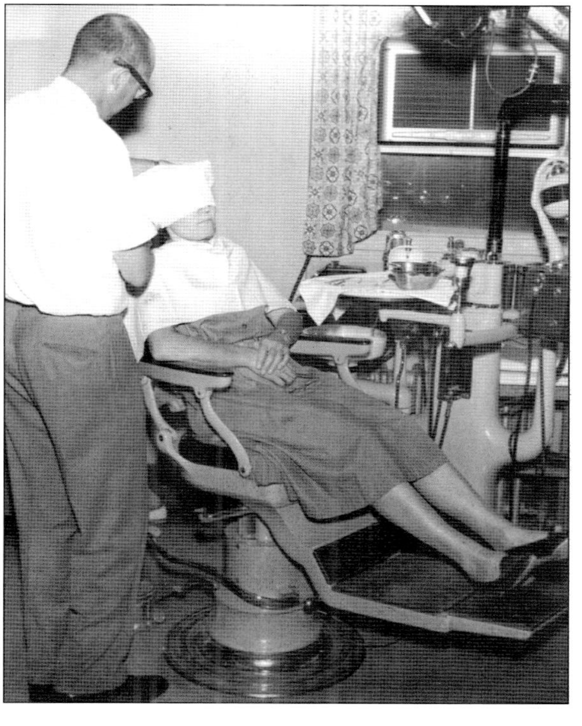

In the 1950s, when Dr. Hayden Donahue was Oklahoma's state mental health director, he implemented a study of the dental needs of patients in mental institutions in the state. Donahue believed that "such a small thing as poor teeth, which kept a patient from eating properly, could add to his mental illness." Consequently, mental institutions in the state set up rooms where a dentist could evaluate the needs of patients. (OHS.)

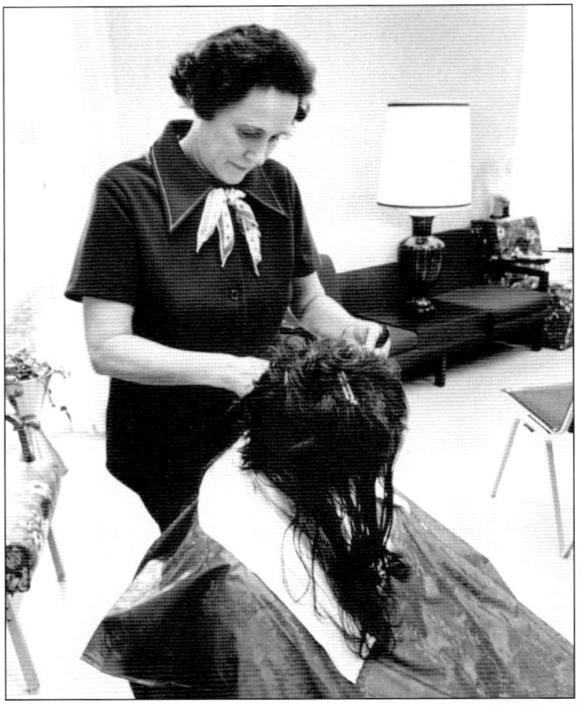

A beauty shop opened in May 1953 at Griffin Memorial Hospital and offered various beauty treatments for female patients. Different volunteer groups raised funds to set up the two-room shop. The volunteers worked under the slogan, "good grooming for mental health." Some of the funds were used to buy cosmetics, hats, purses, and high-heeled shoes. The shop operated for eight hours per day. (OHS.)

In keeping with a new approach to mental wellness, doctors considered vocational therapy a useful tool to help to rehabilitate patients with moderate mental illness. The two men shown here were new patients in the summer of 1954; they took on a project to build a dollhouse. (OHS.)

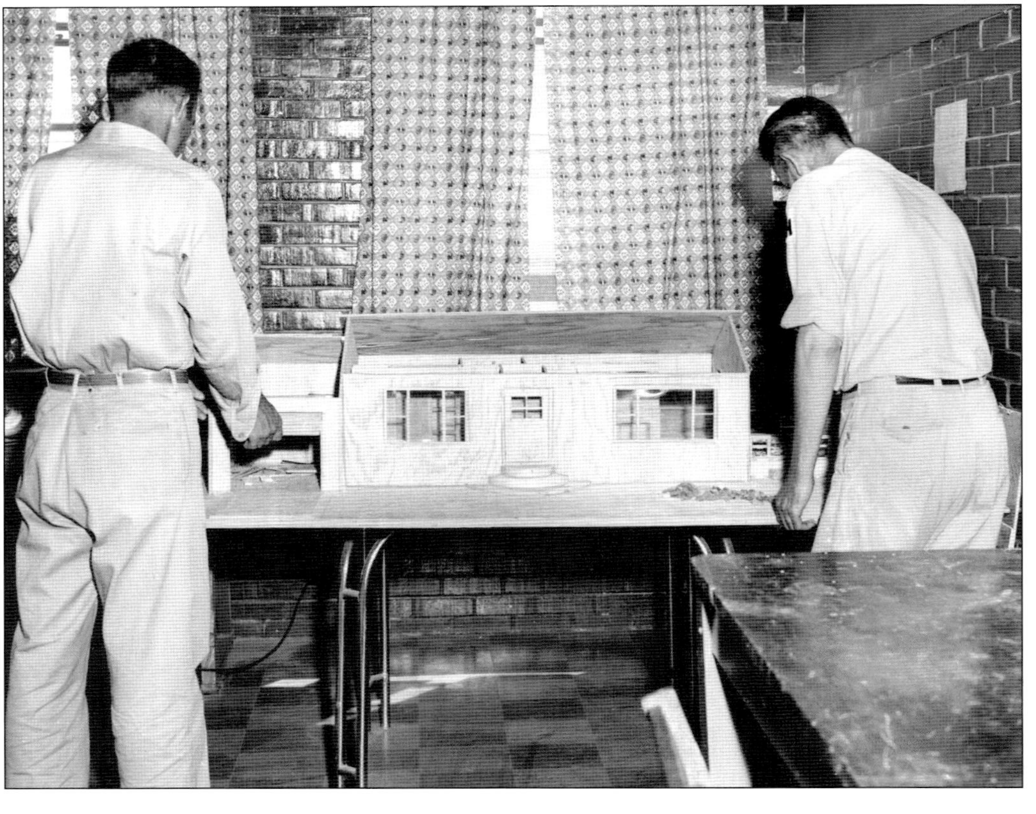

Elderly patients, who made up a majority of the hospital population, were given more recreational opportunities. These opportunities included socializing outside their wards during chaperoned activities like dancing and playing board games. A good portion of the elderly patients were not suffering from mental illness other than the dementia associated with the normal aging process. (OHS.)

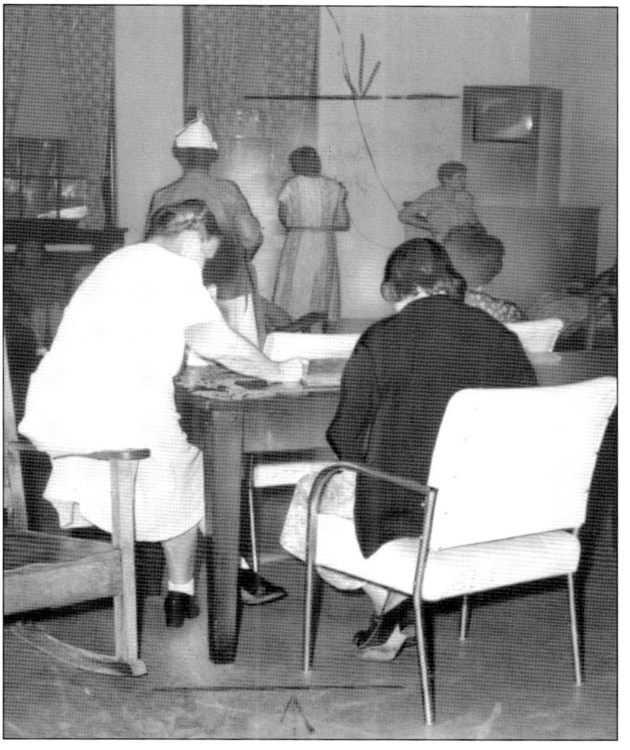

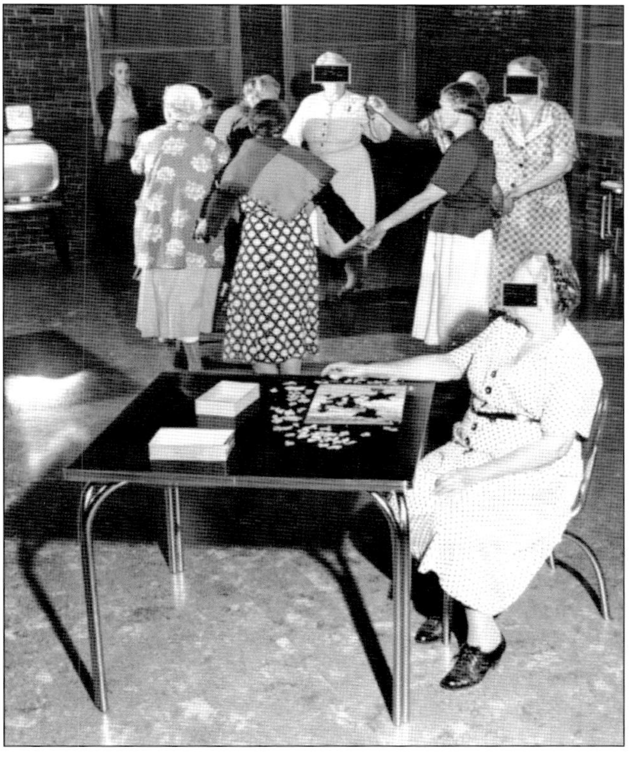

Patients who received shock and insulin therapy and showed improvement were eligible for occupational and recreational therapy. In the late 1940s, the hospital administrator hired two certified occupational therapists who worked with 200 patients per day. As shown in this image, women socialized with other women and worked to solve a puzzle. (OHS.)

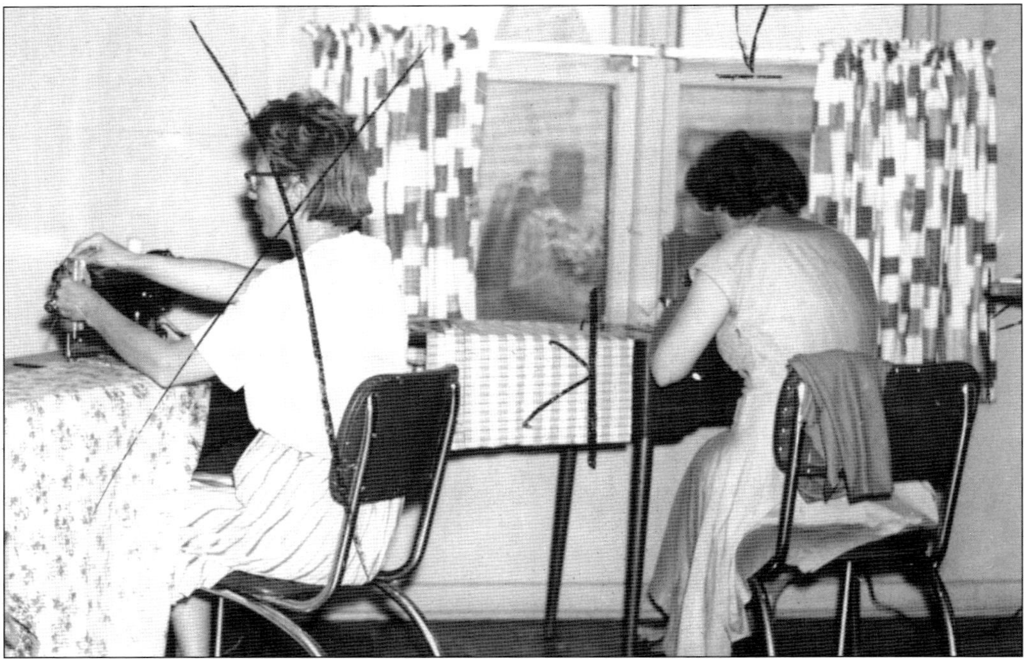

Women were also taught how to sew. The sewing room was one of the more cheerful places in the hospital in the early 1950s. It was decorated with colorful curtains and potted plants. To lift the women's spirits, sewing machines were placed next to windows. (OHS.)

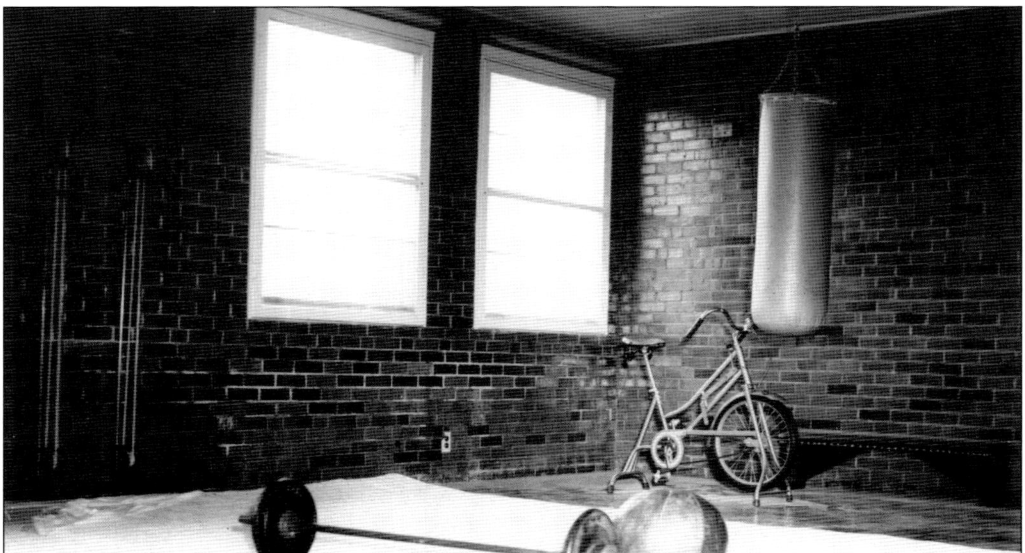

Along with occupational therapy, patients at Griffin Memorial Hospital also had the opportunity to use the exercise room in the gym. Exercise was an important element in a patient's recovery. As shown here, an exercise bar, weights, a punching bag, and a stationary bicycle were available for patients to use. (OHS.)

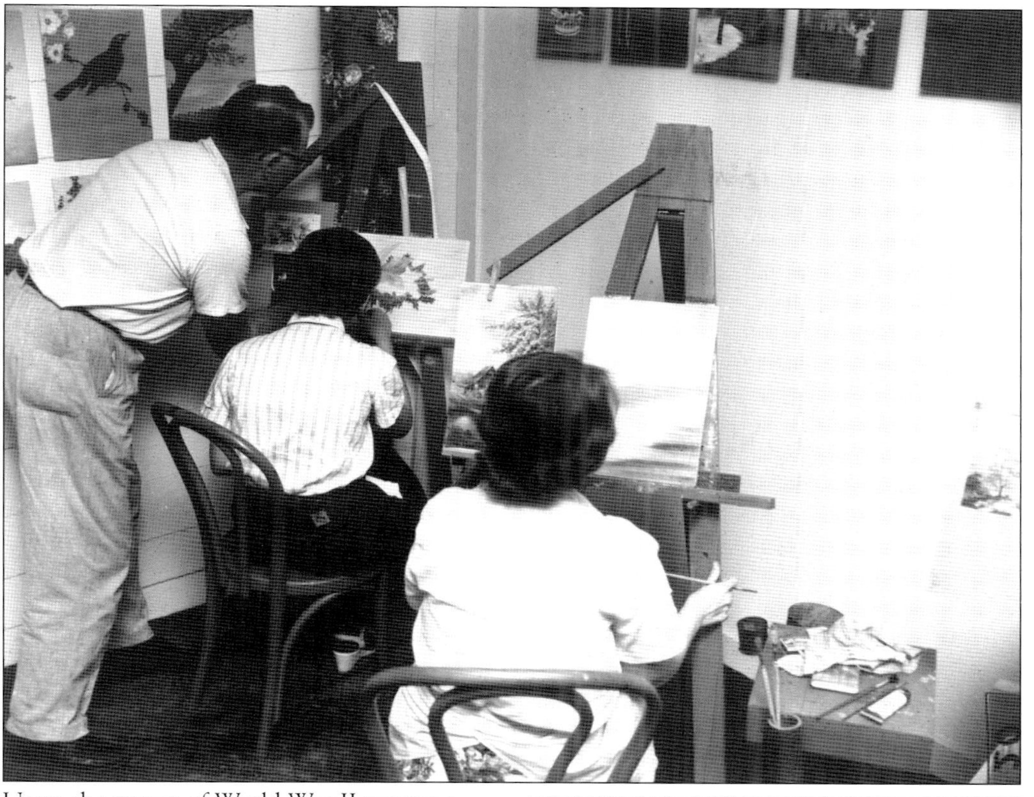

Upon the return of World War II veterans and the recognition by psychiatrists that many of them would need some kind of mental treatment, more and more hospitals and veterans' centers were seeing the benefits of group therapy. Art therapy was one of the tools used with groups for all patients who qualified. Treatment through art expression was first introduced in hospitals as early as the late 1700s. (OHS.)

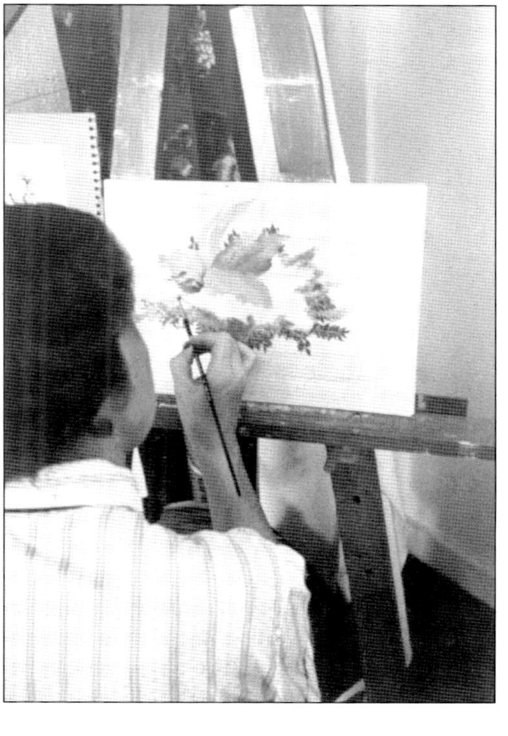

In the 1950s, doctors saw the benefits of artistic expression, but they did not really know how to interpret patient paintings. Doctors tried to study whether paintings revealed something about the patient's symptoms that, in turn, could help the doctors make decisions about their treatments. (OHS.)

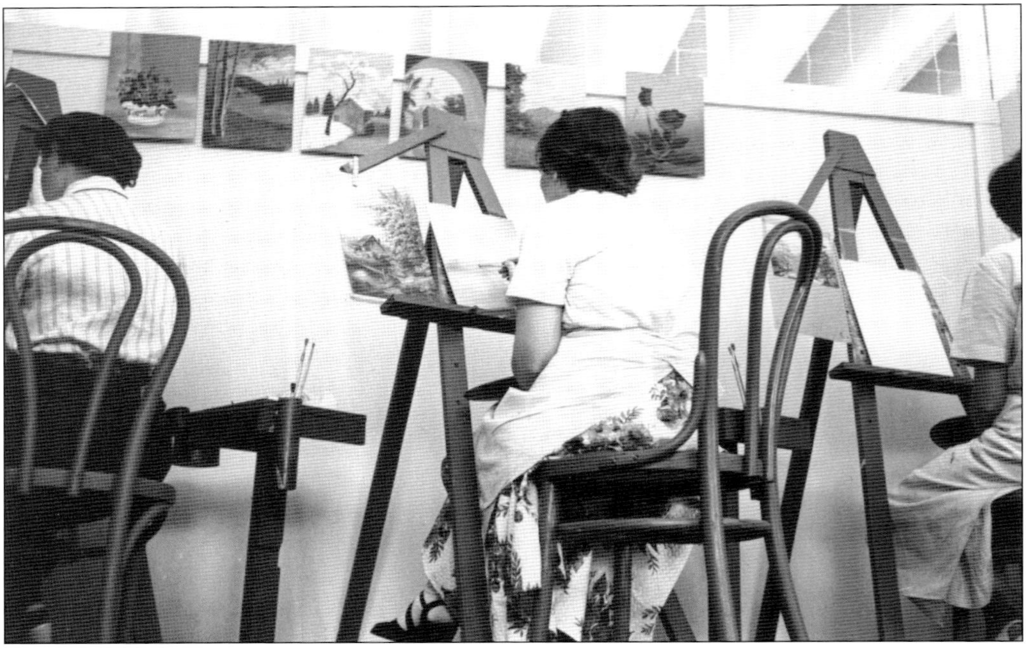

The first art therapists were artists and art teachers. Through observing their students, they began to notice changes in behavior and verbal expression. Later, trained art therapists who believed in the healing influence of a patient's expression on canvas began to consider the medium a "medicine and agent of change," according to therapist Natalie Wallace. (OHS.)

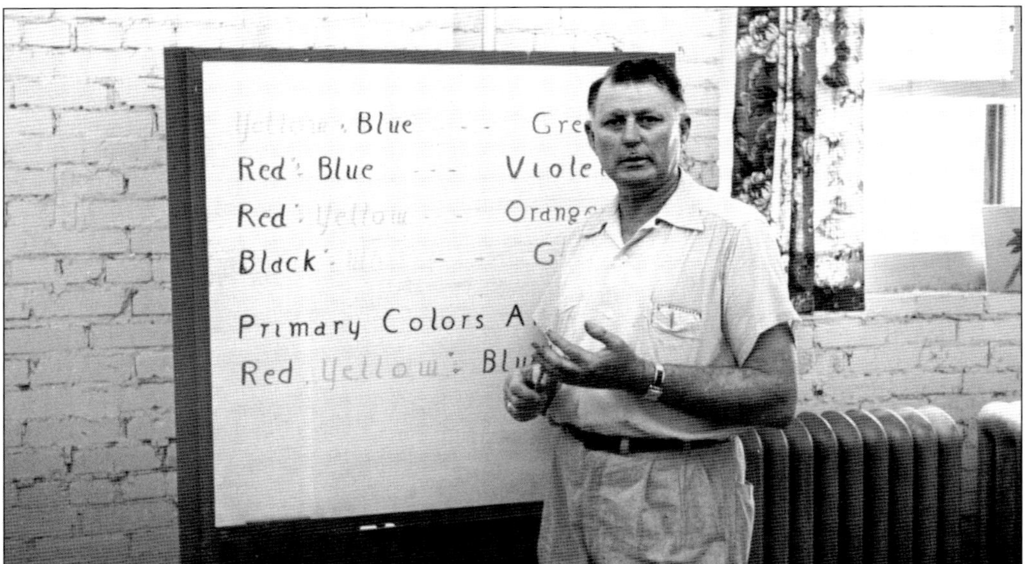

In 1955, Jim Horne became the first person to organize art classes at Griffin Memorial Hospital. Horne, who had studied art at North Texas State University, was employed by the superintendent of Griffin Memorial as an upholster. He noticed that there were patients at the hospital who were bored and had nothing to do. Several of the patients expressed an interest in learning to paint and draw. (OHS.)

Jim Horne talked to the Griffin Memorial Hospital supervisor and received permission to hold a regular art class in 1955. He found a light and airy room to use as a studio. He did not evaluate the paintings, and left it up to students to decide what they wanted to paint. Horne taught two classes on three days each week. (OHS.)

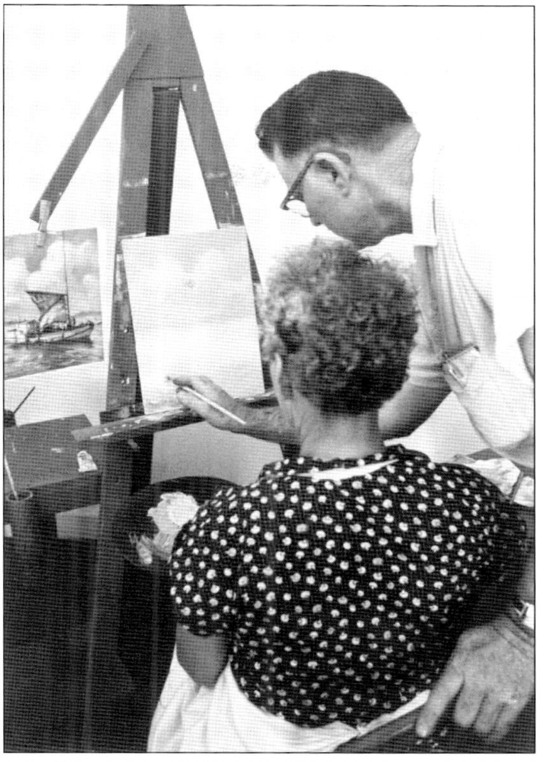

Physicians at Griffin Memorial Hospital believed that Jim Horne's students showed physical and mental improvement after taking art therapy classes. Horne also arranged for patients to have a coffee break during classes; in these breaks, Horne and the patients discussed different aspects of their artwork. With the aid of his students, Horne painted a 14-by-78-foot mural for the hospital's canteen. (OHS.)

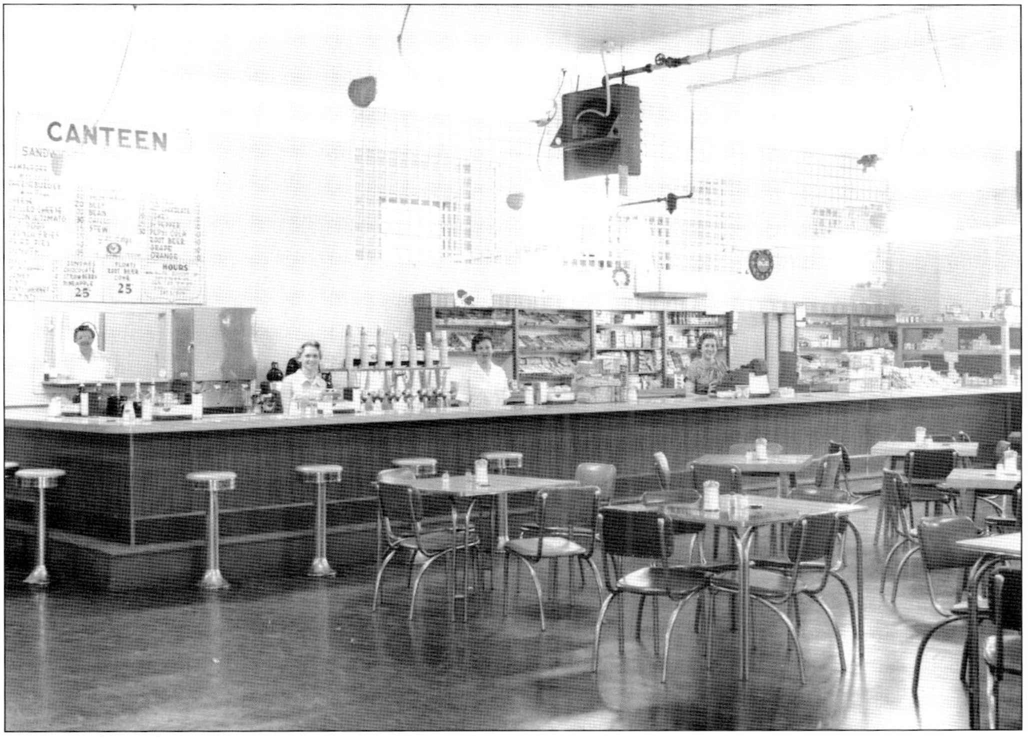

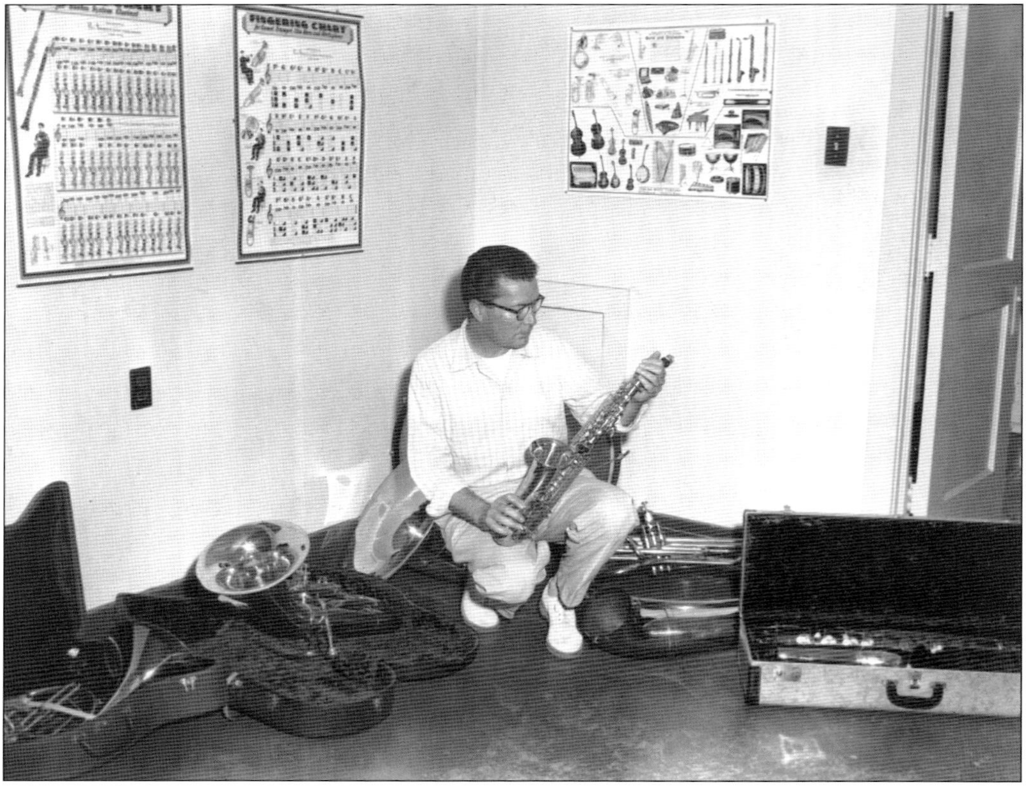

Along with art therapy, music therapy was also offered. The beginning of the music therapy movement in mental hospitals was also recognized as beneficial for veterans who suffered trauma while serving in World War II. Music was seen as a treatment for depression and replaced a reliance on psychological, pharmacological, and other such therapies. (OHS.)

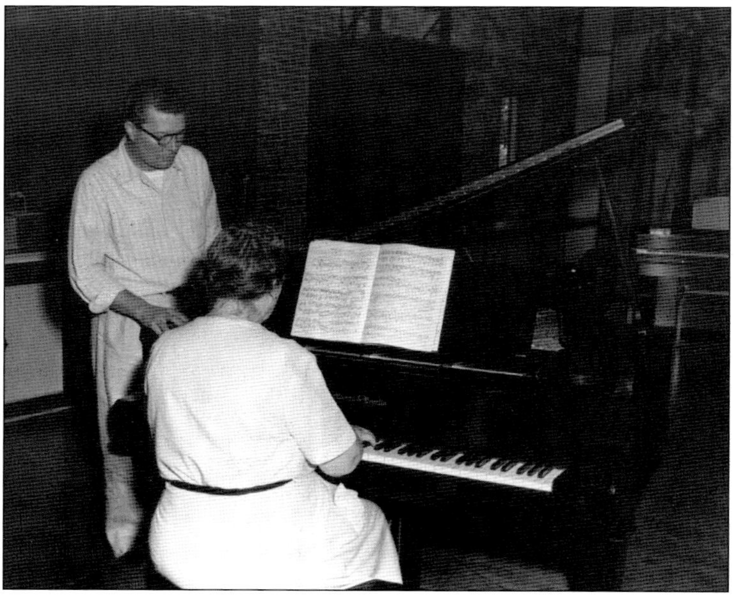

In 1944, Michigan State University became the first university to establish a music therapy program in its school of music. Music's benefits to mental patients was different than those provided by art therapy. In the 19th century, it was thought that music reached deep into the soul of the patient. Those who taught music therapy were educated in psychiatry and psychotherapy. (OHS.)

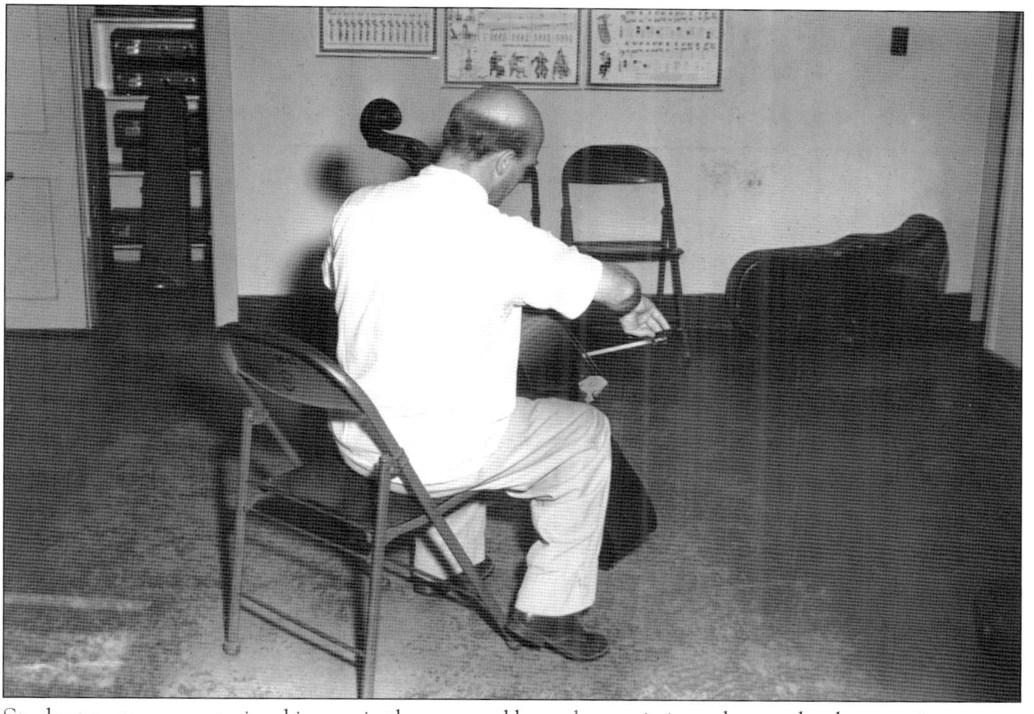

Student nurses were trained in music therapy and brought music into the wards where patients were managed and had very little energy. When these patients saw the nurses dancing to the music, they began to join in. The patients' reaction to music encouraged the creation of programs for them that included learning how to play musical instruments and classes in music appreciation. (OHS.)

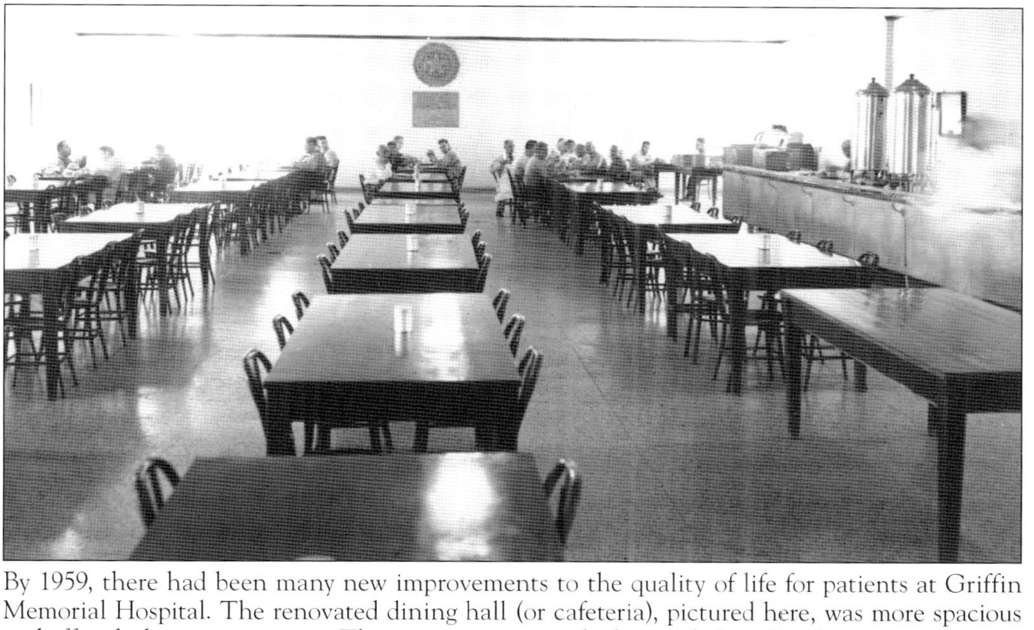

By 1959, there had been many new improvements to the quality of life for patients at Griffin Memorial Hospital. The renovated dining hall (or cafeteria), pictured here, was more spacious and offered a better experience. The improvements to the hospital also offered more employment opportunities for citizens of Norman. (OHS.)

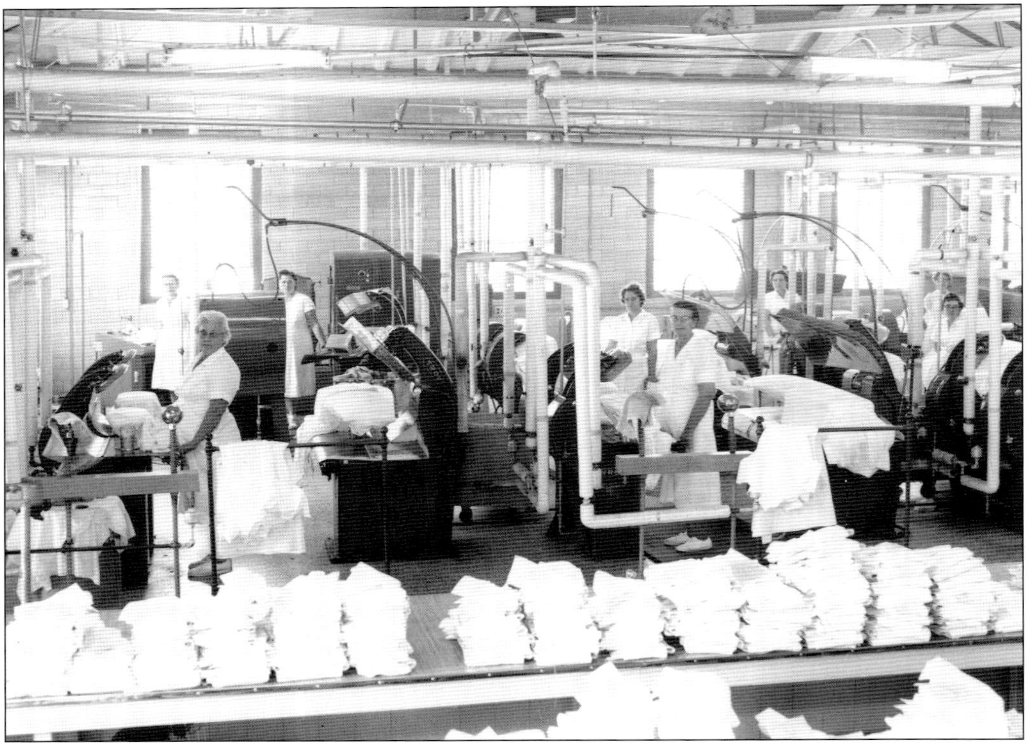

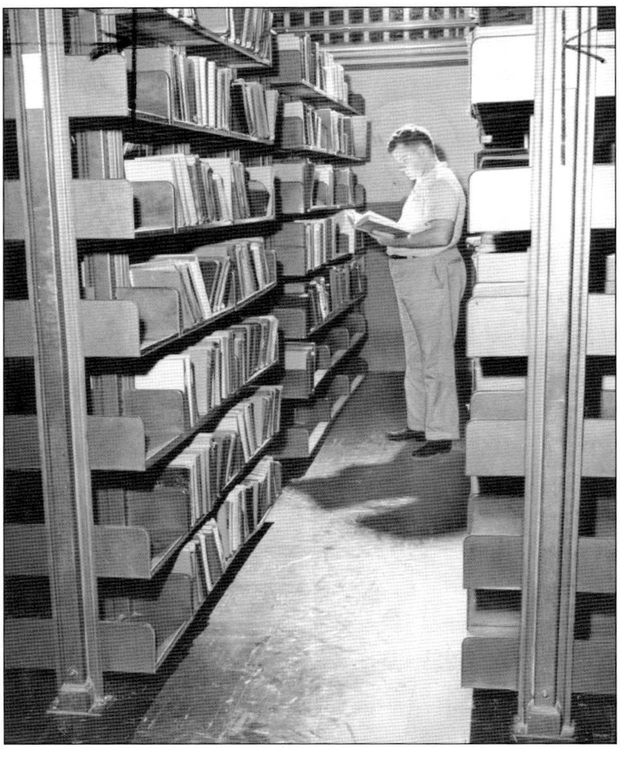

In the 1950s, a new laundry was completed at Griffin Memorial Hospital. This provided employment for citizens of Norman and patients at Griffin Memorial. The new laundry had a larger capacity and made it possible for patients to have clean clothes every day. (OHS.)

In 1958, there were 900 employees working at Griffin Memorial Hospital in positions ranging from library clerk to farm manager. In the 1940 census, the hospital only had 87 employees, and a majority of those were attendants. In the 1950s, the hospital was one of Norman's major employers, with positions that included switchboard operator, dairyman, occupational therapist, record manager, and dietitian. Most of the employees lived in Norman. (OHS.)

Six

The Era of Dr. Hayden Donahue

1960s

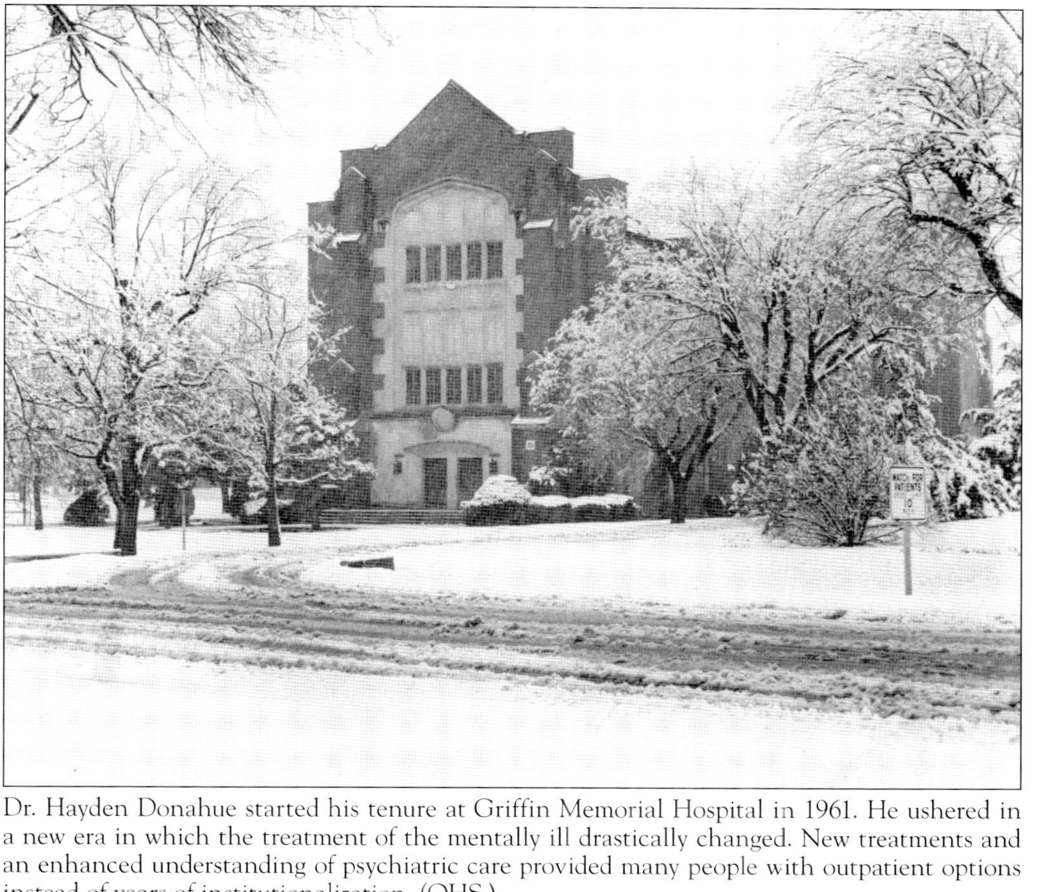

Dr. Hayden Donahue started his tenure at Griffin Memorial Hospital in 1961. He ushered in a new era in which the treatment of the mentally ill drastically changed. New treatments and an enhanced understanding of psychiatric care provided many people with outpatient options instead of years of institutionalization. (OHS.)

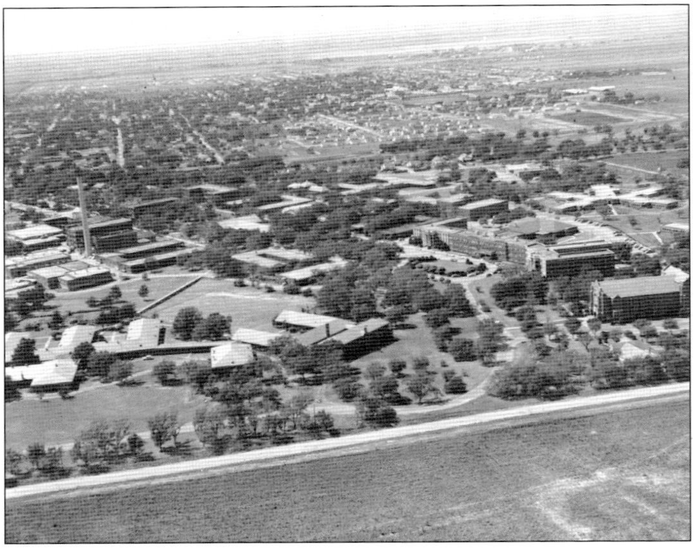

The facilities at Griffin Memorial Hospital expanded in the 1950s because of an increase in state appropriations and the implementation of modern techniques in the care of the mentally ill. However, the 1950s would be the last decade when superintendents sought state financial aid to alleviate overcrowding and insufficient medical staff. A new way of treating mental illness that emerged in the late 1950s and 1960s helped to make institutionalized care nearly obsolete. (OHS.)

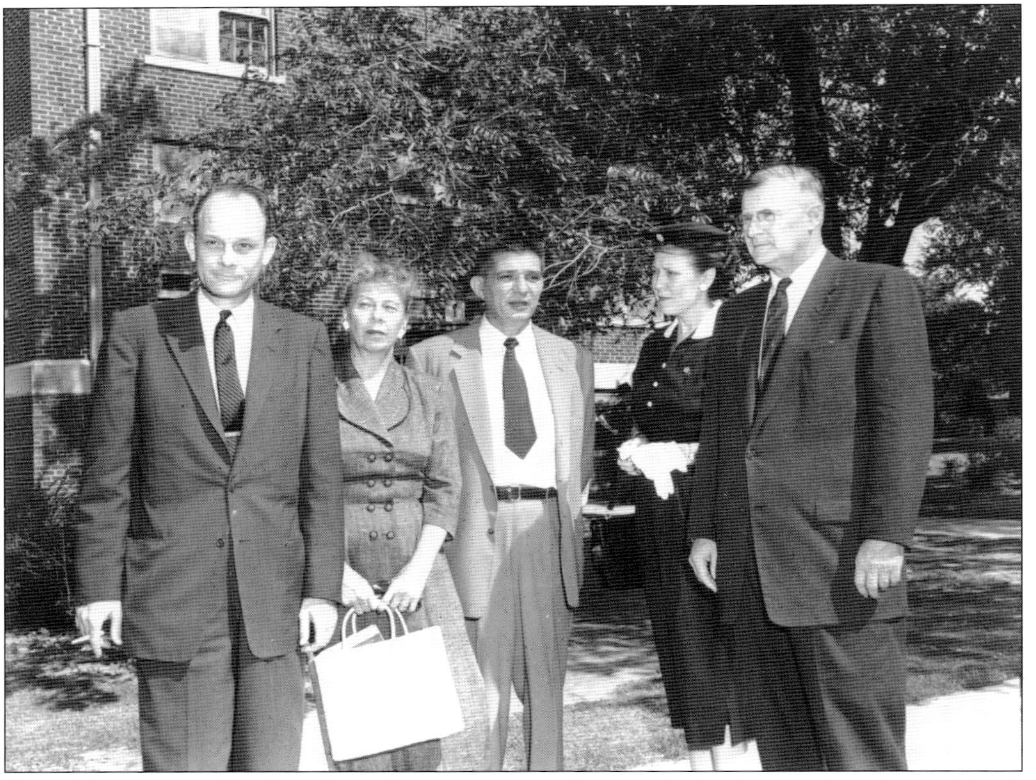

One of the impacts of Dr. Donahue's time as superintendent was his implementation of a psychiatric residency program and the establishment of a children's ward. He also was one of the main proponents of federally funded community mental health centers, which changed institutional treatment programs to focus more on outpatient care. Griffin Memorial's new buildings in the 1960s included a vocational rehabilitation center and a community health care center. Donahue is pictured here at far left. (OHS.)

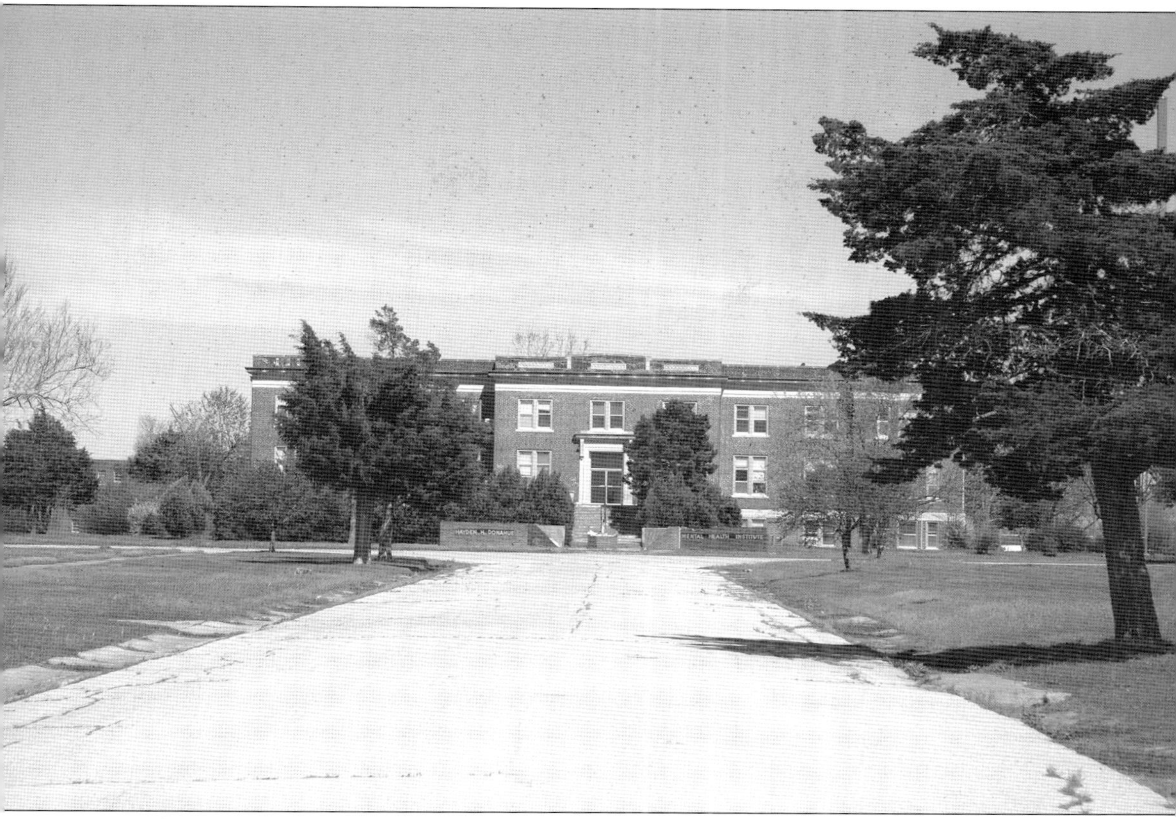

Dr. Donahue's belief that community centers for the mentally ill would help to deinstitutionalize the mental health care system came from his service in North Africa during World War II. While there, Donahue worked with a psychologist, Roy Grinker, to help soldiers who suffered from combat stress. The success rate of returning soldiers to a healthy life was 43 percent better than the rate of success during and after World War I. This convinced Donahue that some of those with some forms of mental illness did not have to be in institutions. After the war, Donahue worked in Gen. Omar Bradley's office in Washington, DC, to redevelop the Veterans Administration. Later, Donahue worked in Little Rock, Arkansas, where he helped develop state homes for the mentally Ill. While he was in Arkansas and Texas, Donahue helped draft mental health laws for those states. Pictured here is the Hayden N. Donahue Mental Health Institute in 2020. (CCHS.)

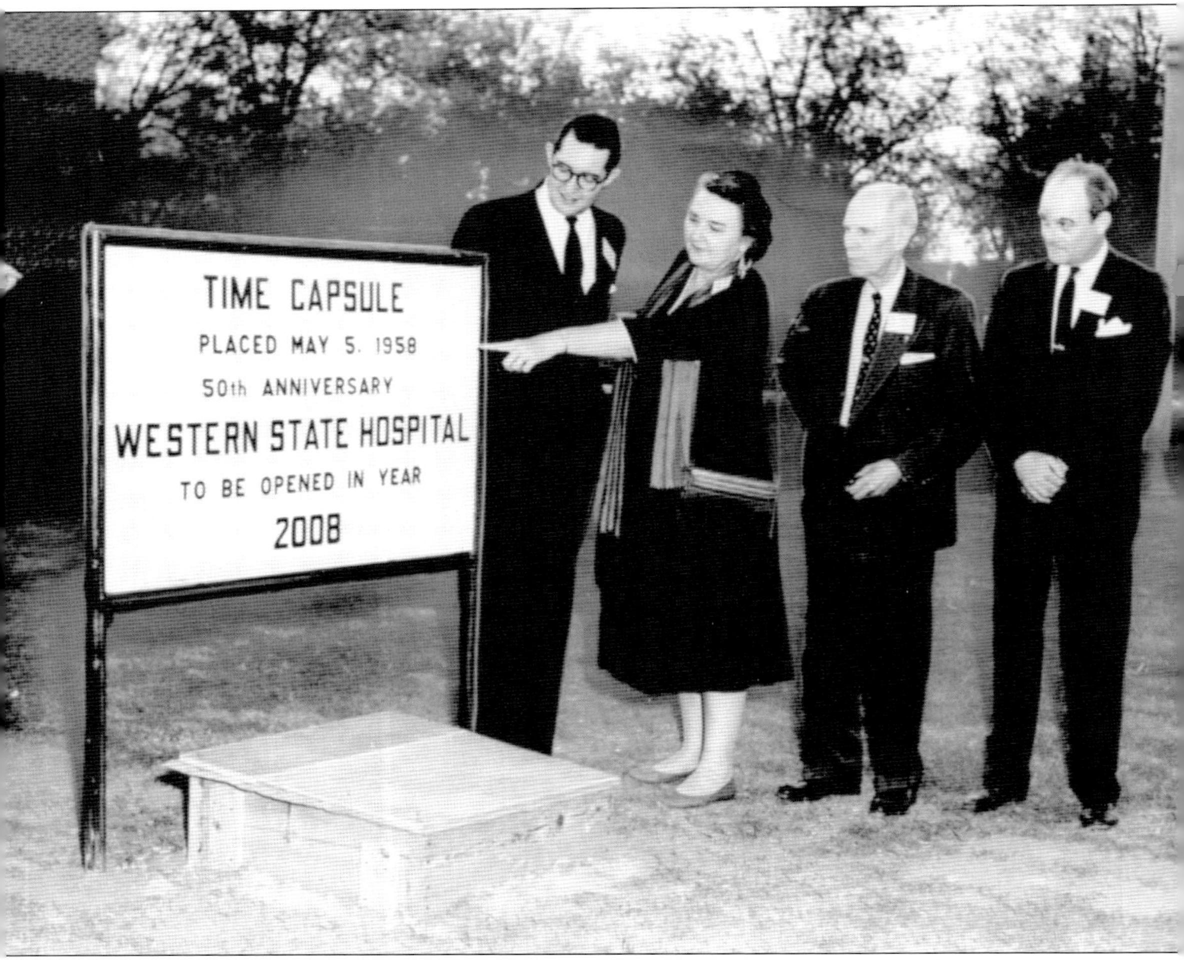
TIME CAPSULE
PLACED MAY 5. 1958
50th ANNIVERSARY
WESTERN STATE HOSPITAL
TO BE OPENED IN YEAR
2008

Dr. Donahue was asked by the Oklahoma legislature to come to the state to help draft mental health legislation. He became the first director of Oklahoma's Mental Health Department. With his exceptional qualifications, Donahue was the ideal person to take over as superintendent at Griffin Memorial in 1961. When Donahue (far right) took over as superintendent, he brought a different approach to treatment and held a different philosophy in the relationship between mental health and spiritual health. He stated that the "real attainment of man's maturity comes when he is able to find ultimate meaning for his existence." Donahue maintained that most people with emotional problems sought the guidance of a minister. He believed that it was important for ministers to recognize when a person with emotional problems needed professional psychiatric help. Donahue also advised that the New Testament provided many examples of Jesus taking on the role of therapist in working with people around him. (OHS.)

During Dr. Donahue's tenure as superintendent of Griffin Memorial, he advocated for the construction of a children's ward that was completely independent from adult patients. When Donahue assumed his position in 1961, the hospital was the only state facility for mentally ill children. Under his leadership, a new ward was built for children. (OHS.)

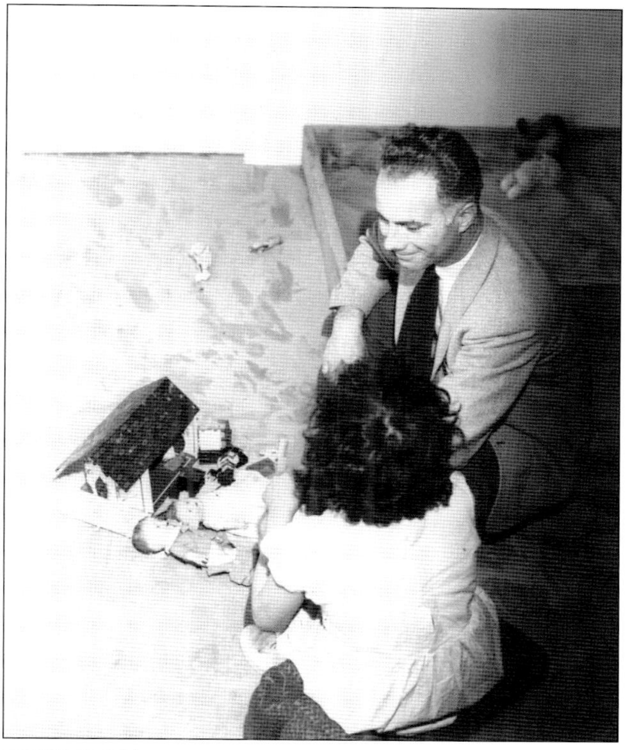

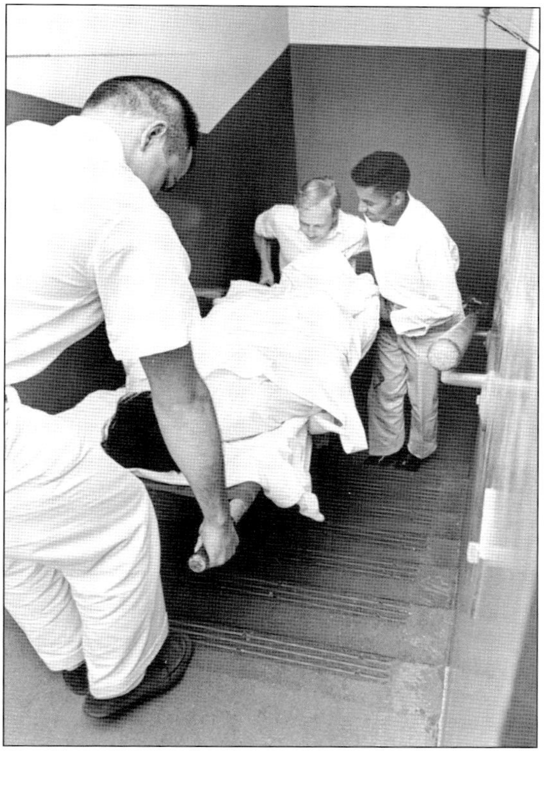

In 1965, Dr. Donahue campaigned to promote an election for a $54 million state bond, which was on the ballot in the December 15, 1965, election. After the bond passed, Griffin Memorial Hospital's allocation was $2,998,255 for improvements. Along with funding the construction of a new children's ward, part of the money went toward the instillation of four new elevators that would eliminate the need for attendants to have to maneuver patients through stairwells, as shown here. (OHS.)

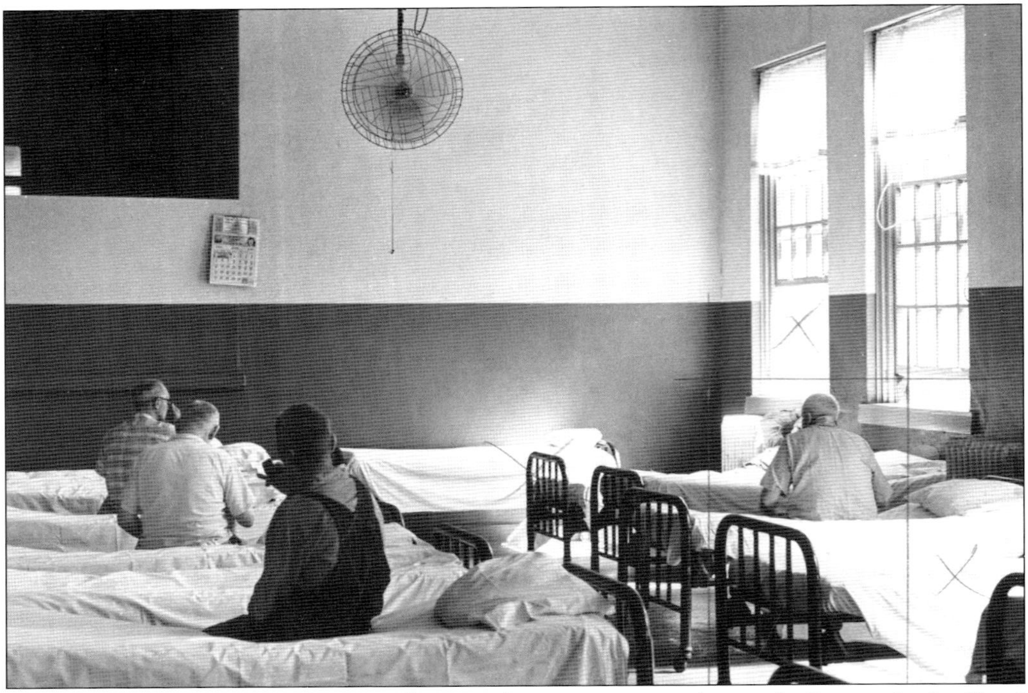

The 1965 bond also was used to install air-conditioning units in the wards. Patients had suffered for decades in wards with poor ventilation, which doctors believed was a detriment to their recovery. The misery of Oklahoma summers was first alleviated with fans; air-conditioning was a welcome addition for the comfort of both patients and staff. (OHS.)

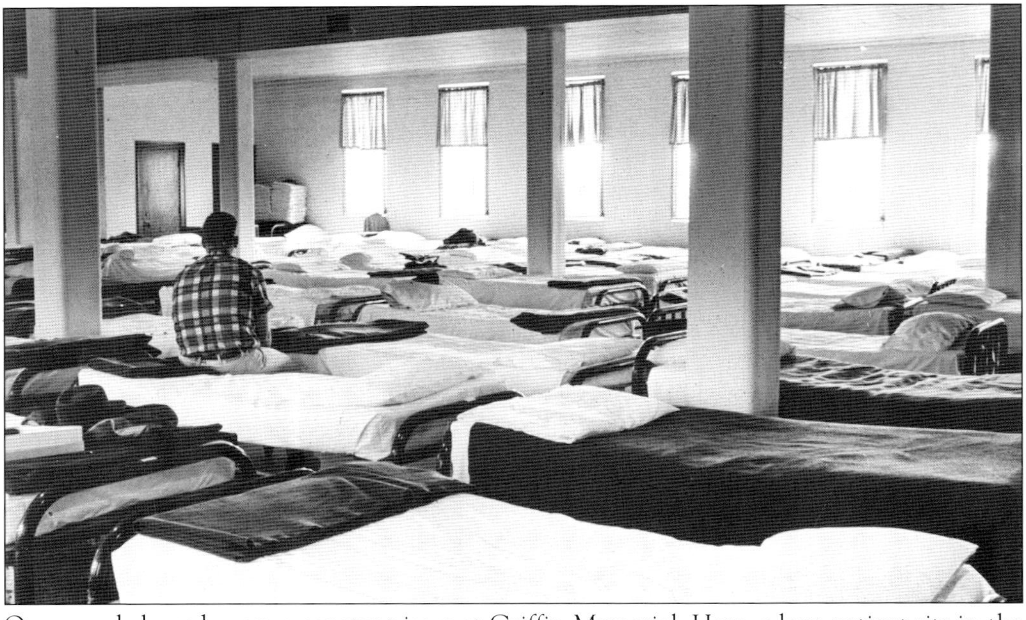

Overcrowded wards were a constant issue at Griffin Memorial. Here, a lone patient sits in the crowded sleeping area of his ward. Some of the funds from the $54 million state bond that passed in 1965 were used to build more partitioned cubicles to provide some privacy for patients. (OHS.)

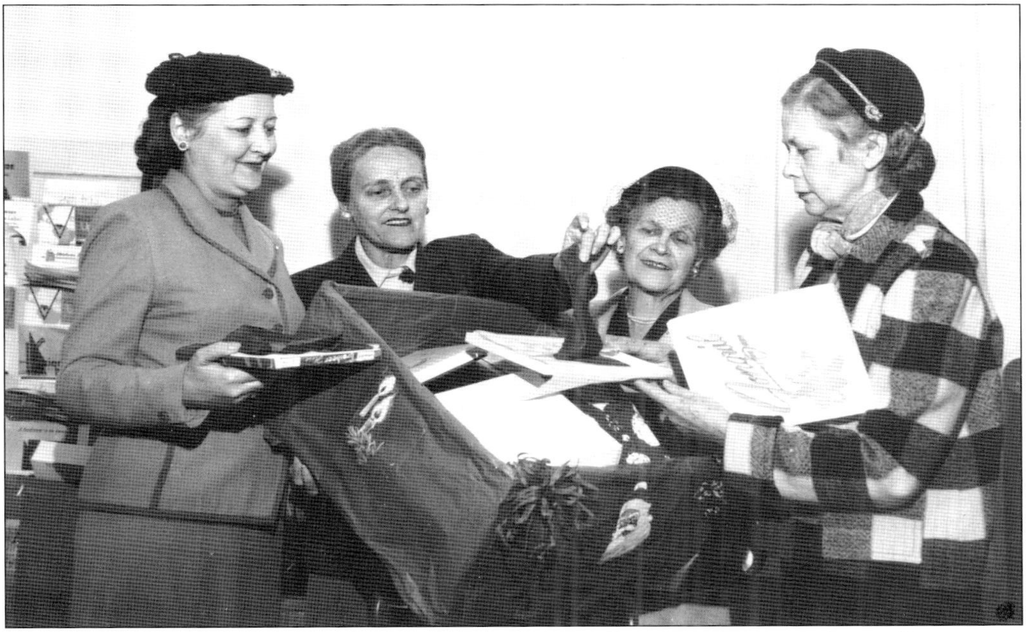

Clubs and volunteer groups found Christmas to be a perfect time to express their willingness to provide patients with Christmas gifts. Here, women in the Hospital Auxiliary and University of Oklahoma's Panhellenic organization prepare gifts for patients at Griffin Memorial. (OHS.)

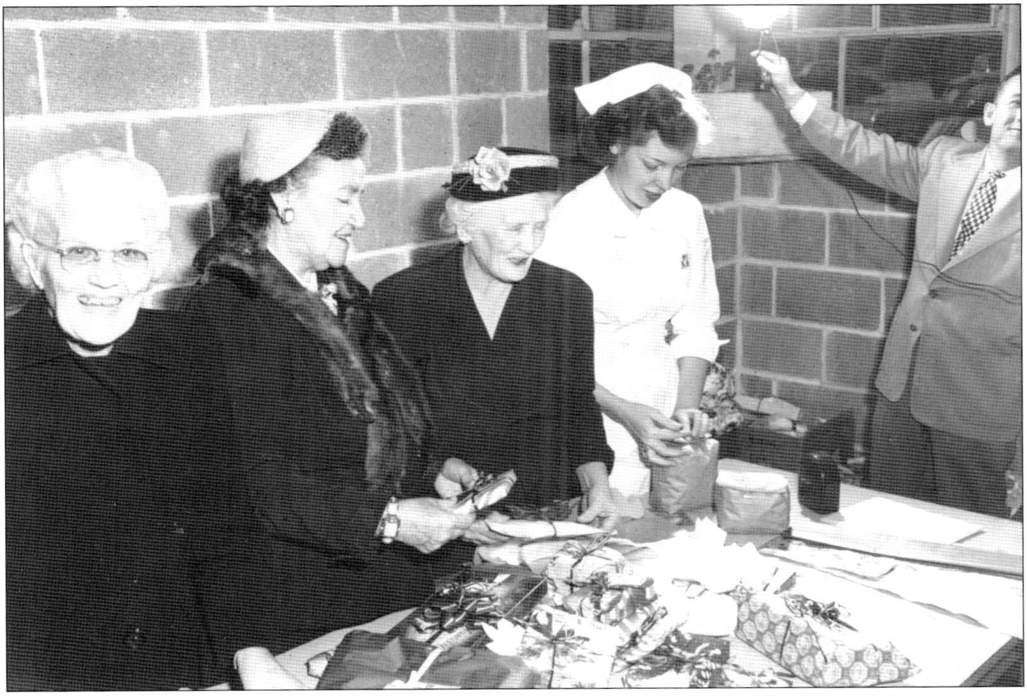

Norman's garden clubs also held Christmas parties. Each club donated gifts and candies. One garden club provided a doll dress to one of the patients whose doll did not have a dress; this club decided that their goal would be to supply dolls and clothing for Christmas gifts. (OHS.)

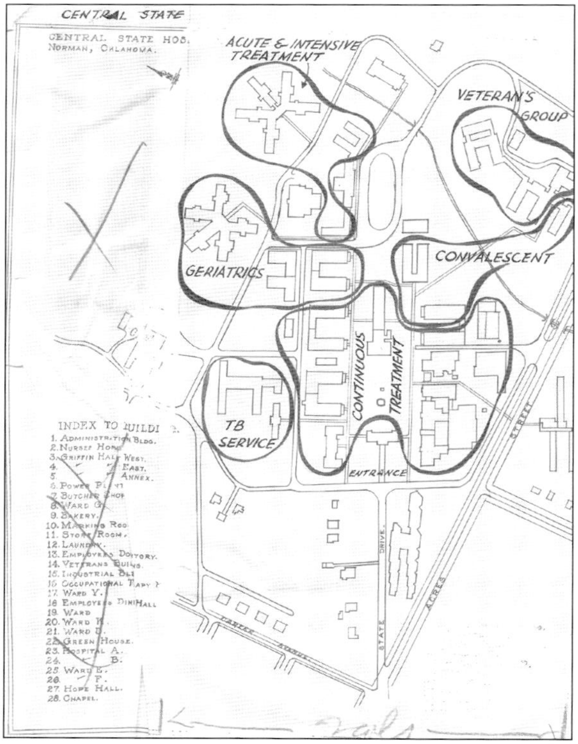

As shown on this 1953 map, Central State Hospital designated facilities according to a certain criterion of care. As early as 1958, one option intended to help patients move from continuous treatment to complete recovery was a halfway house. The facility held 10 to 15 patients who learned the social and occupational skills needed to resume lives outside the hospital. (OHS.)

Two buildings constructed around the same time occupied an area behind Hope Hall. At upper right is the farm at the corner of Robinson Street and Twelfth Avenue. The building at center was designated for geriatric patients and was constructed in 1952. (OHS.)

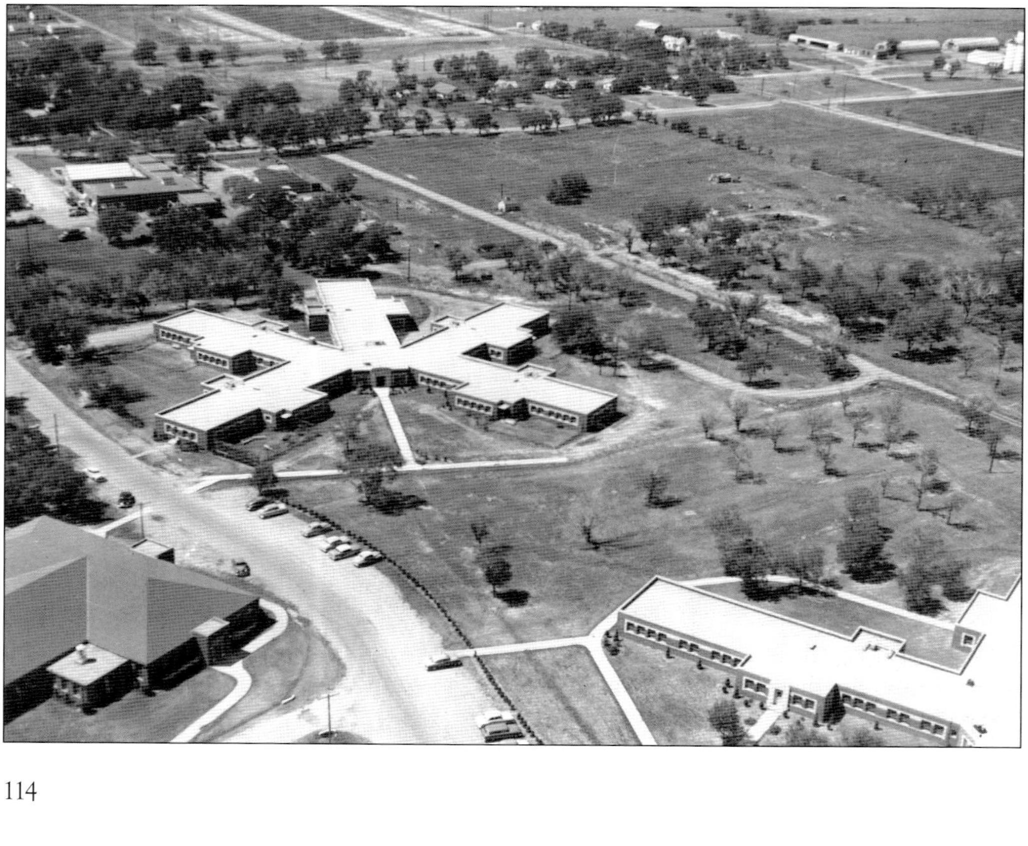

The entrance to the geriatric compound had a misspelling in the carved stone. As one newspaper report stated: "Sculptor Neat but his spelling's poor, as doctors point out at Central State Hospital, Norman, where the sculptor got his 'I' and 'A' transposed when this building was erected in 1952 for elderly patients." (OHS.)

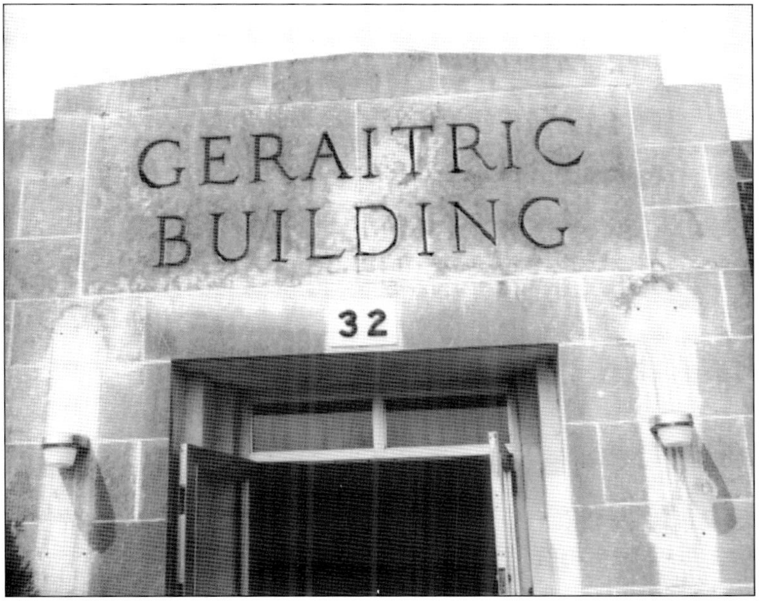

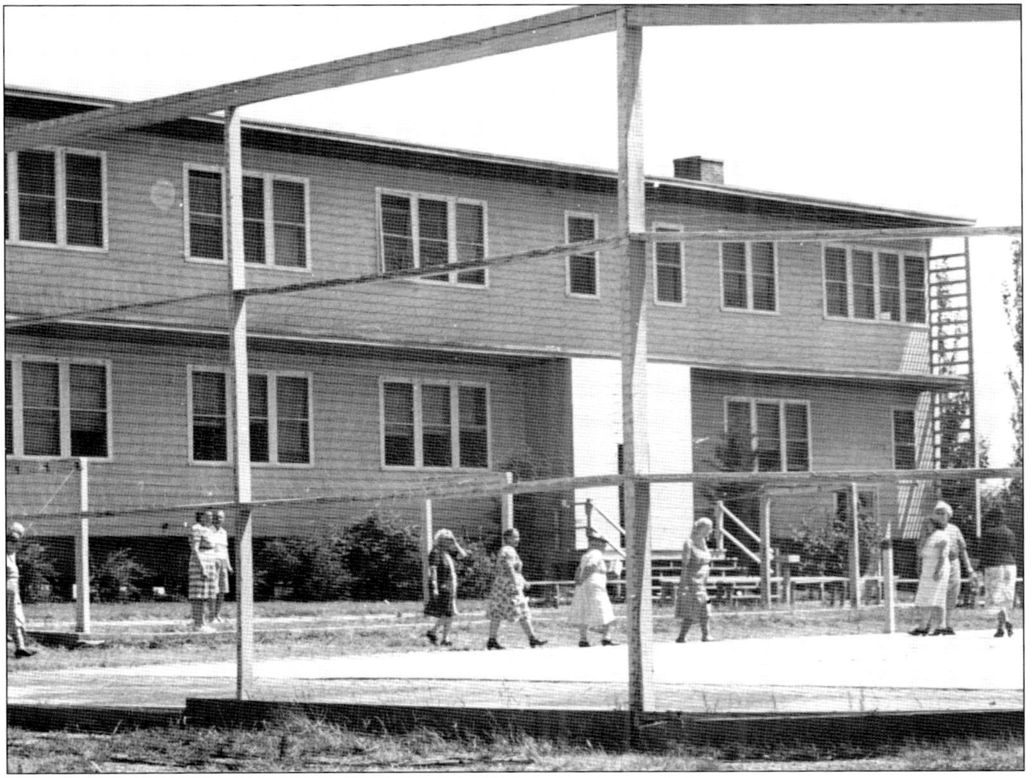

When *Daily Oklahoman* reporter Mike Gorman investigated the conditions at Central State in 1946, he noted that the only recreation for older women was a fenced area where they were allowed to walk around and enjoy the sunshine. There was basically no other recreation for the elderly. (OHS.)

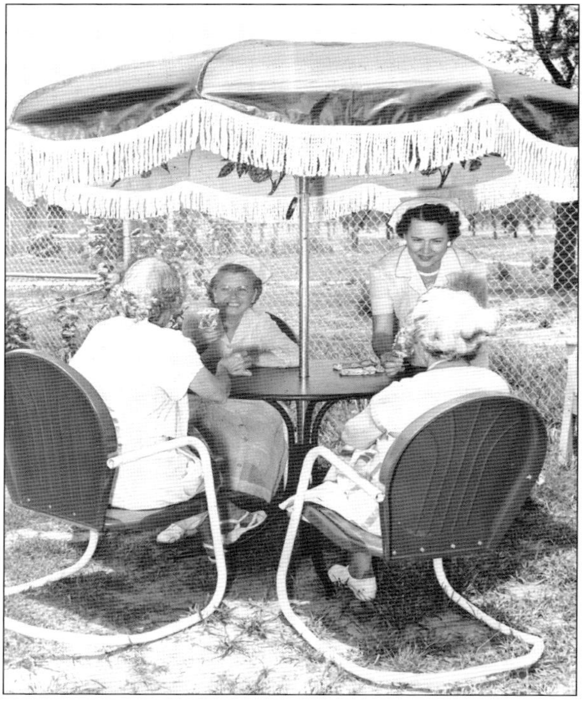

An isolated geriatric ward and area for elderly patients was prominent in 1958. The goal was to offer surroundings for older patients that did not limit their quality of life, as had been the case with their confinement in the 1940s. In this 1953 photograph, two elderly women are shown trying out the new "beach set." (OHS.)

A ward for acute care was built east of the geriatric ward, most likely around 1952. This aerial photograph shows the acute care facility directly behind the east end of Hope Hall. Today, there is only an empty field there. (OHS.)

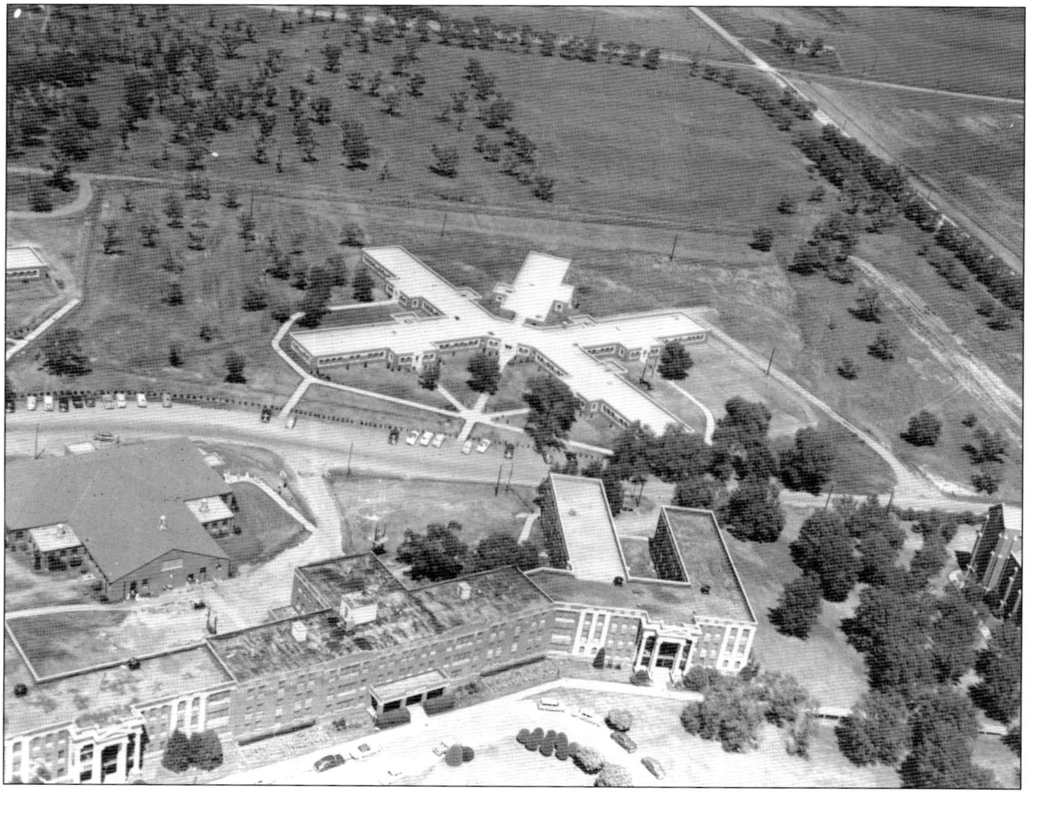

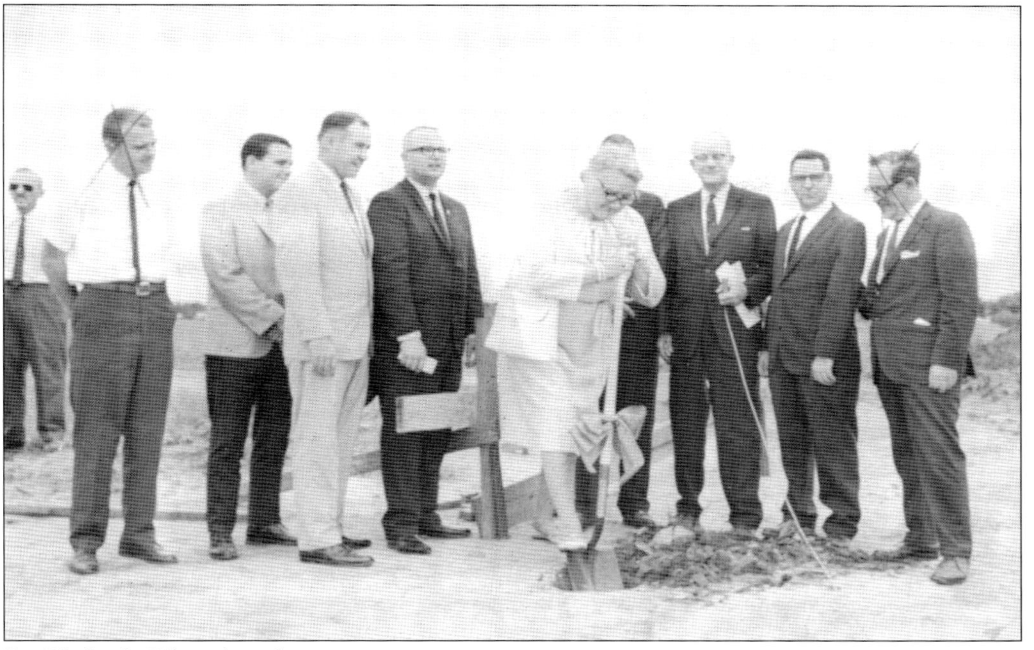

Dr. Rheba L. Edwards is shown breaking ground for a new vocational rehabilitation center in 1963. The $760,000 center was a joint effort between the hospital and the vocational rehabilitation division of the Oklahoma State Department of Education. The vocational center replaced the halfway house concept and served more patients in their efforts to gain the skills they needed to resume living outside of the hospital. (OHS.)

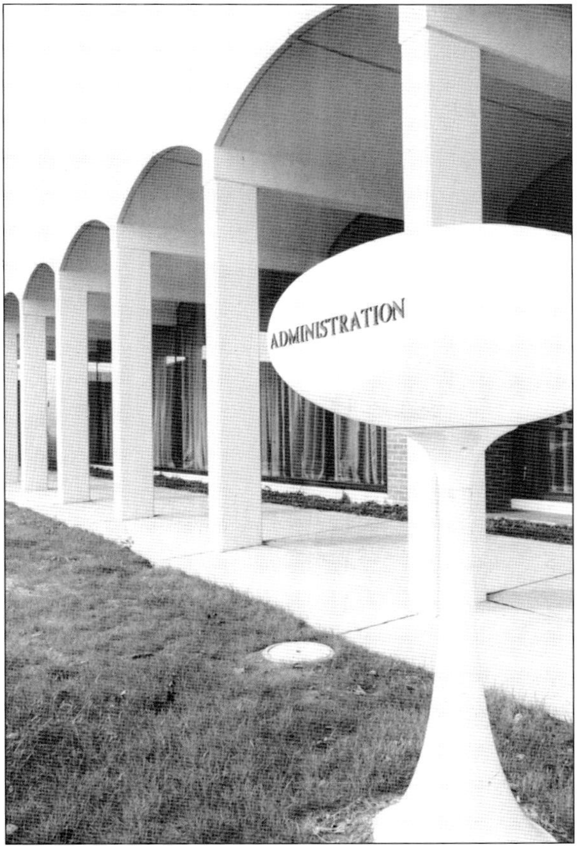

Dr. Edwards, director of rehabilitation and aftercare at Griffin Memorial, stated that the purpose of the vocational rehabilitation center was to help patients "approach the problems of normal life." At the vocational center, patients underwent job tolerance through industrial therapy before they were released. Job tolerance was encouraged through working in the laundry or the cafeteria. (OHS.)

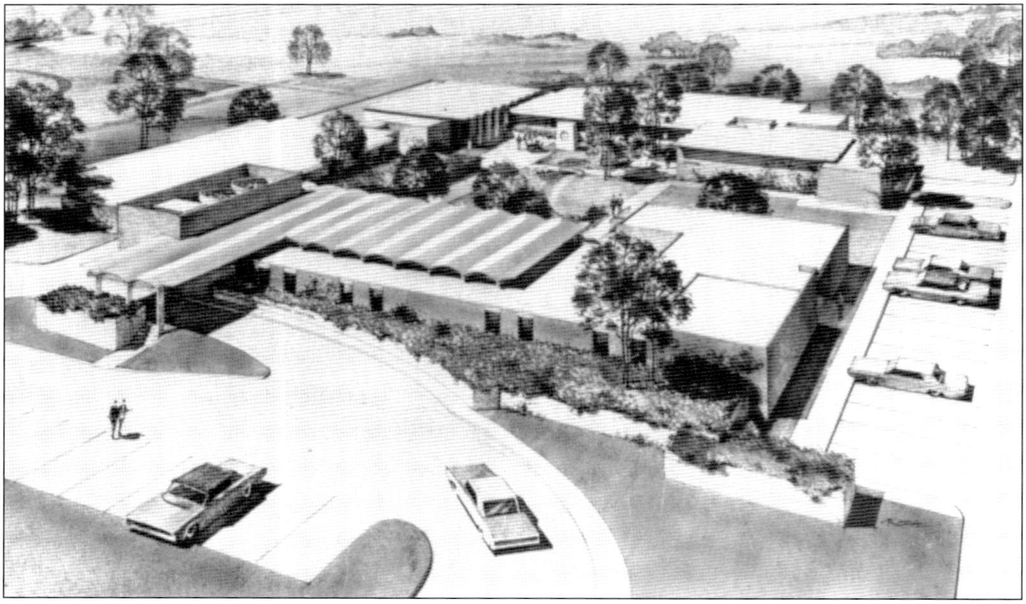

Dr. Hayden Donahue, who served as superintendent at Griffin Memorial from 1961 to 1979, was one of the principal draftsmen of federally funded community mental health and rehabilitation centers. The centers presented a new treatment option for patients who had mental problems that were not severe enough for the person to be confined to a mental institution. Pictured is one of several architectural renderings of a rehabilitation center at Griffin Memorial. (OHS.)

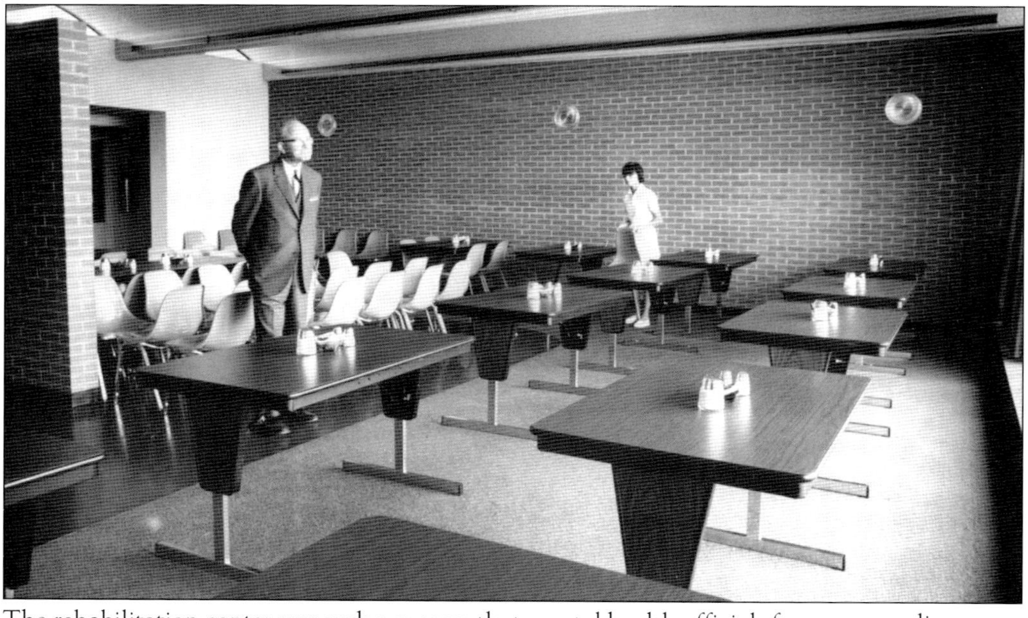

The rehabilitation center was such a success that mental health officials from surrounding states visited Griffin Memorial to ascertain if the same program would work in their state. A group of visitors from Nevada and Missouri stated that they believed the rehabilitation center at Griffin had a good teaching program and were impressed with the relationship between the hospital and the rehabilitation center. (OHS.)

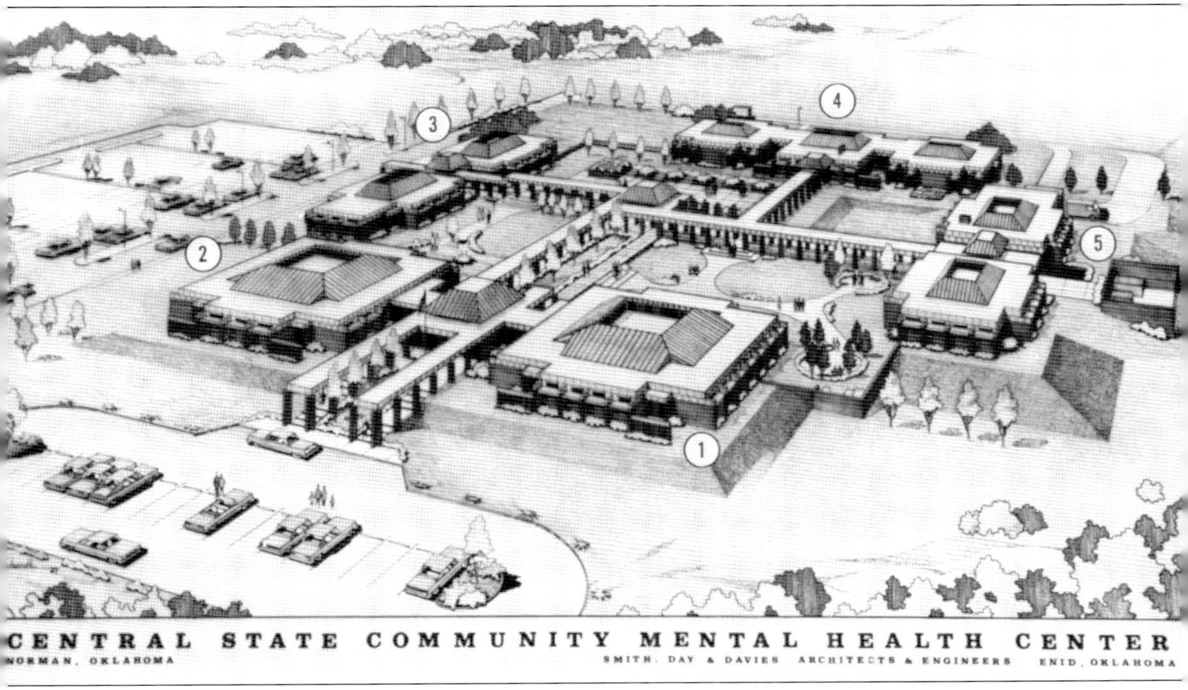

The move to deinstitutionalize patient care at Griffin Memorial and treat patients on an outpatient basis came to fruition when Dr. Donahue promoted the creation of a community health care center. Donahue fought for this concept for many years, and by 1967, his plan had been brought to life in this architect's drawing, which shows a multiuse complex connected by covered walkways. Today, this facility is on the south end of Griffin Memorial Hospital property and faces Alameda Street. In 1969, Building 1 housed outpatient services. Building 2 housed a day hospital. Occupational therapy services were provided at the back of Building 2. Inpatient services were offered in Building 4, at the north end of the property. Building 5 contained dining services. The $1 million center was approved by the Oklahoma legislature, with $750,000 provided by the federal government. (OHS.)

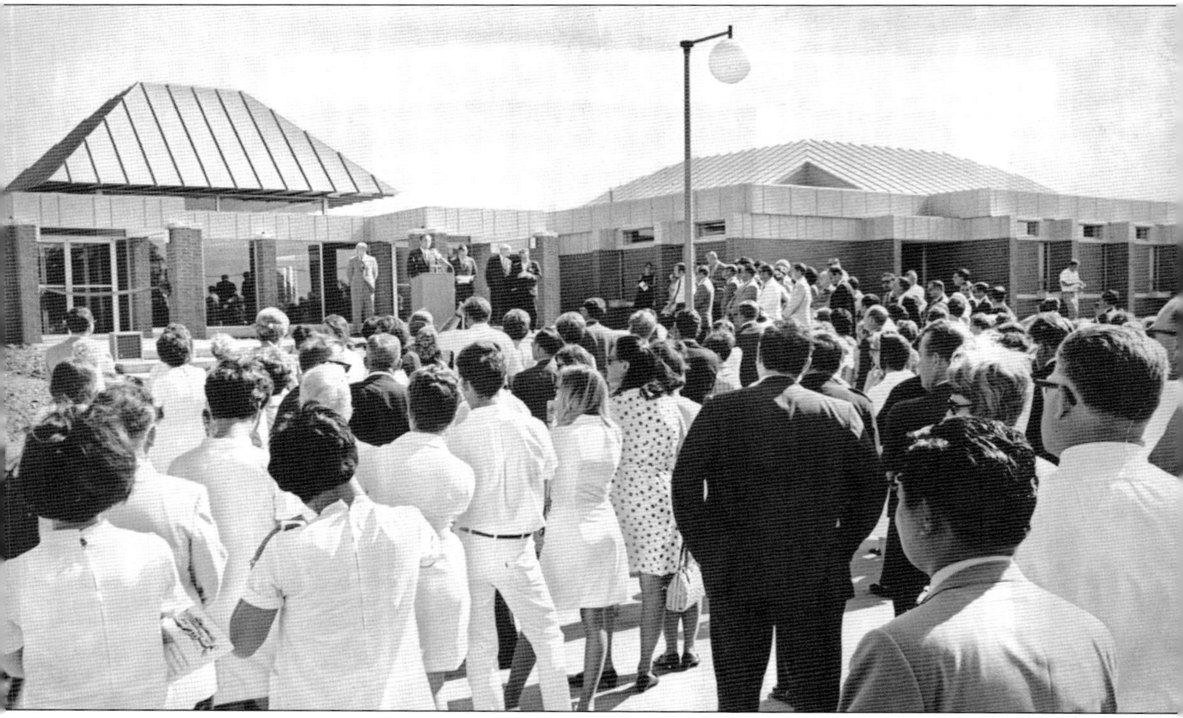

In 1969, the long-awaited community mental health care center opened on the grounds of Central State Griffin Memorial Hospital. At the time, the center was considered one of the most progressive treatment centers in the country. A new phase in treatment started with Dr. Donahue's efforts to treat most cases of mental illness on an outpatient basis. However, there were problems for some patients who had been housed at Griffin for decades. These patients were considered treatable and were transitioned by professional staff into mainstream society. But many had no place to go, and did not transition successfully. These patients considered the hospital their home. The outside world was alien to them. Thanks to the efforts of Donahue and other advocates of deinstitutionalization, the maintenance of the old asylum, building more wards to alleviate overcrowding, and the state paying to take any sort of care of mentally ill patients became a thing of the past. (OHS.)

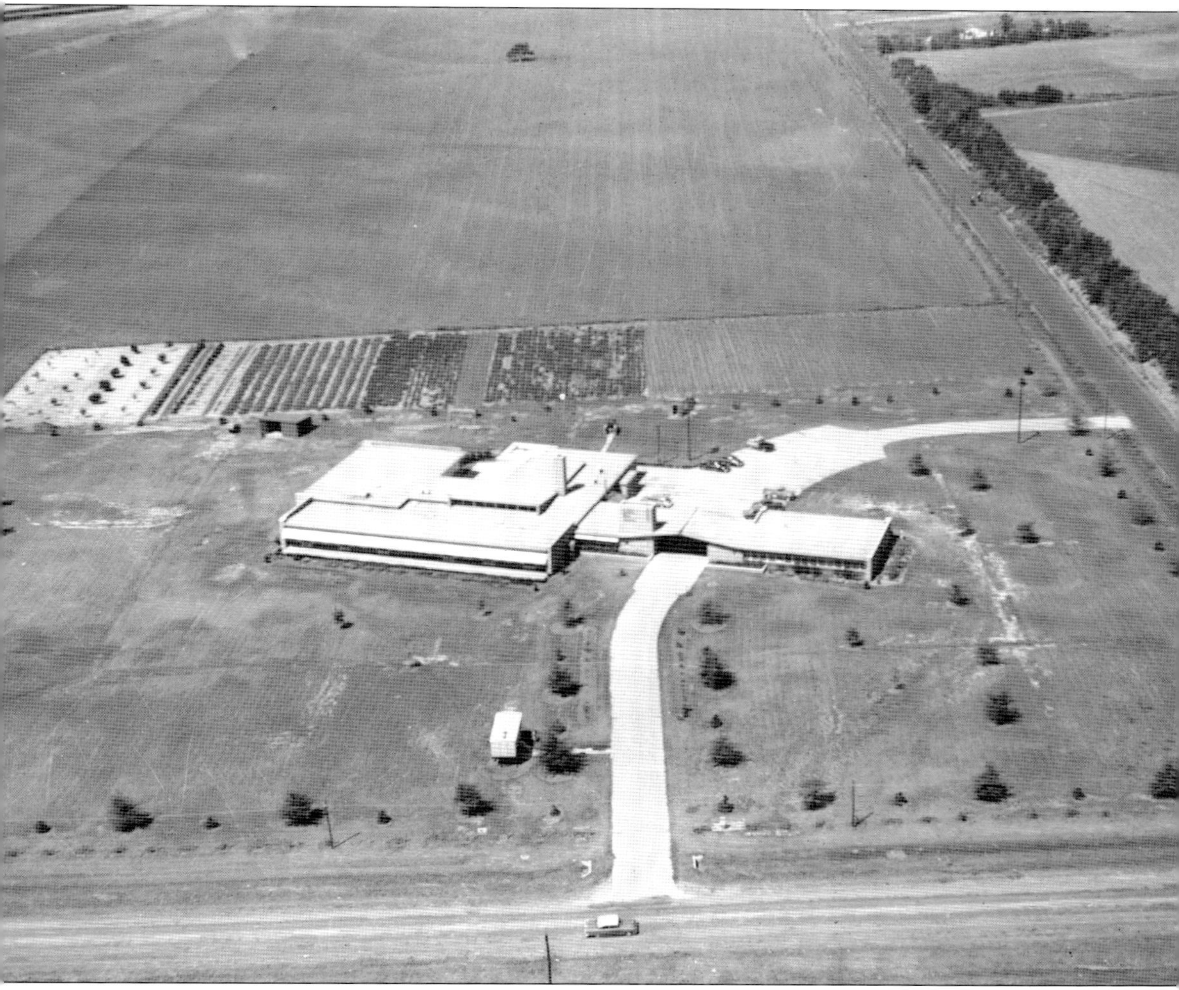

In 1955, the Oklahoma Cerebral Palsy Institute was on the northeast corner of Griffin Memorial Hospital property at Alameda Street and Twelfth Avenue. The center began in 1946, when the national honor society of the American Legion voted to create a facility that would offer intense therapy and schooling for children. The facility was referred to as the Charitable Spastic Institute for Children. Spastic paralysis referred to a lack of muscular coordination. The American Legion was responsible for the cost of personnel and equipment. The institute was one of four in the country and was the only one that was charitable; the other three were private. Initially, the center opened with four children and one nurse. Each week, another child was admitted until the total reached 16. The training lasted for three to six months. The institute suggested that parents continue the training at home. (OHS.)

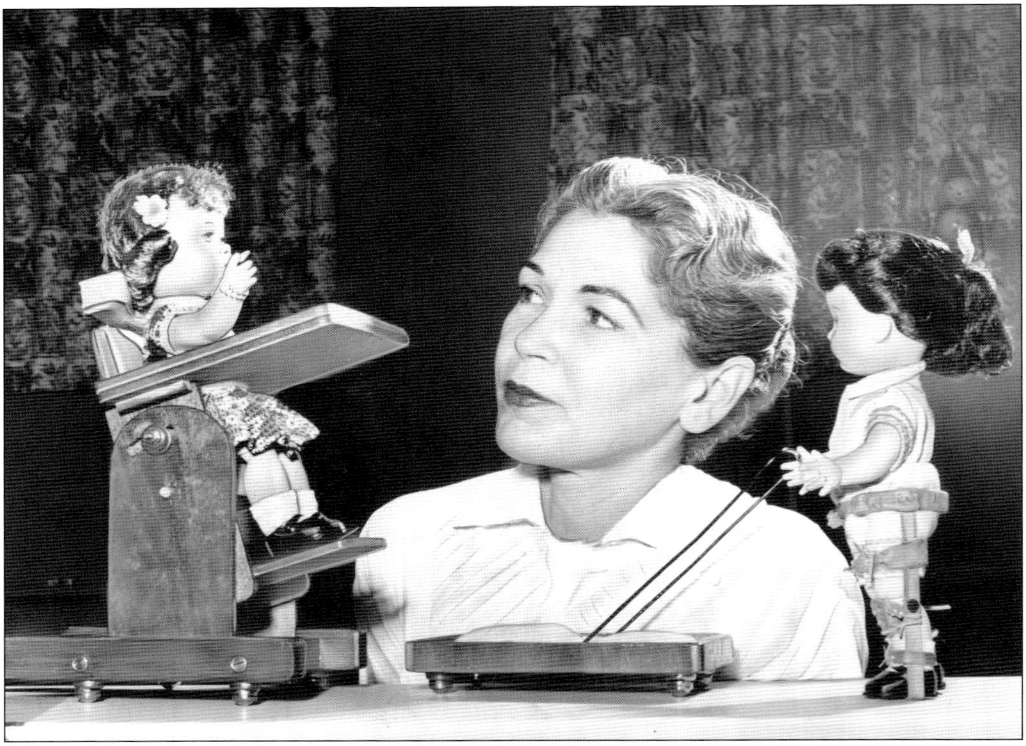

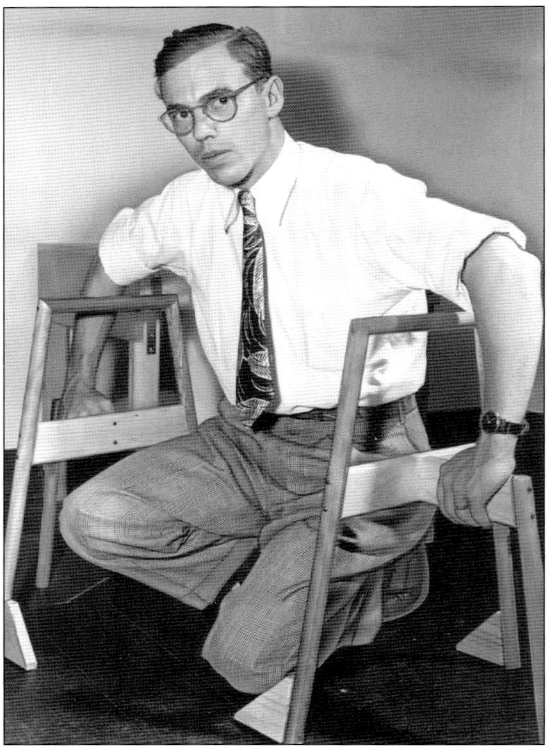

In 1948, the Charitable Spastic Institute for Children, located at the former naval base (South Base) changed its name to the Cerebral Palsy Institute. From 1948 to 1953, state legislators sponsored legislation to build and fund a facility to house the institute. Pictured is Bettie Ward, an occupational therapy aide at the institute. (OHS.)

In 1953, the Cerebral Palsy Institute moved to 1125 Alameda Street on the southern part of state-owned property. Donald J. Hess, administrative director of the Cerebral Palsy Institute, is displaying specially designed crutches that were part of the new equipment used in the treatment of cerebral palsy patients. (OHS.)

A tradition started in the 1950s at Griffin Memorial Hospital involving students from various organizations volunteering time to help at Griffin Memorial and the Cerebral Palsy Institute. Young patients are pictured here with University of Oklahoma sorority members. The program at the institute included occupational and physical therapy along with speech correction. (OHS.)

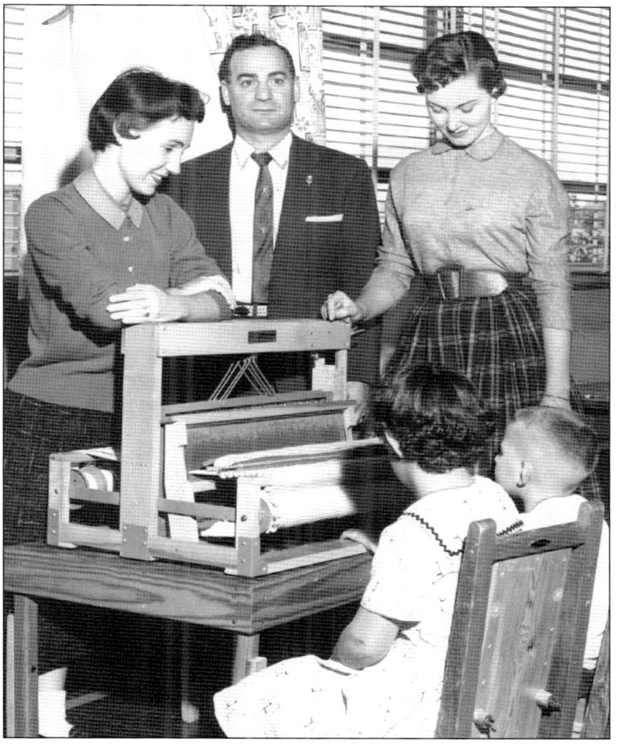

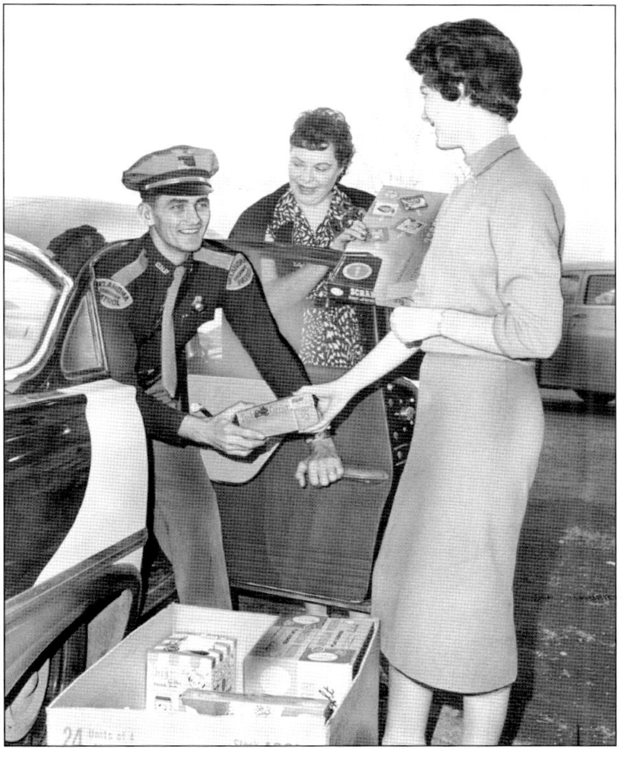

The source of cerebral palsy is thought to be a brain injury that might have occurred during pregnancy or a premature birth in which the fetus did not receive enough oxygen or other nutrients. Children at the institute were not forgotten. Employees from the Oklahoma Department of Public Safety are shown unloading gifts for children at the Cerebral Palsy Institute. (OHS.)

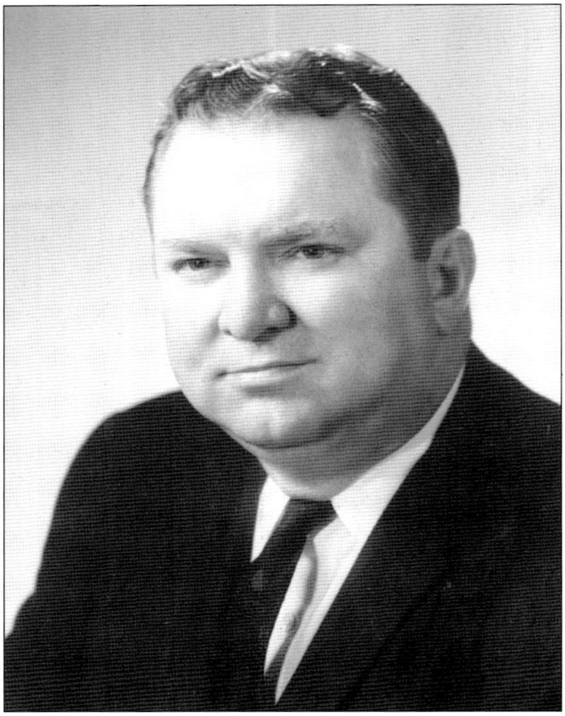

In 1981, the Cerebral Palsy Institute was renamed the J.D. McCarty Center for Children with Developmental Disabilities. McCarty was first elected to the Oklahoma House of Representatives in 1940, and served three terms as speaker of the house; he died in 1980. (OHS.)

In this picture taken at the J.D. McCarty Center for Children with Developmental Disabilities, Timothy Hopkins (age seven) tries out a tricycle while being watched by Ron Martin (center), president of the Sooner AMBUCS (American Business Clubs) Norman chapter, and Curt Peters, chief executive officer of the J.D. McCarty Center. (OHS.)

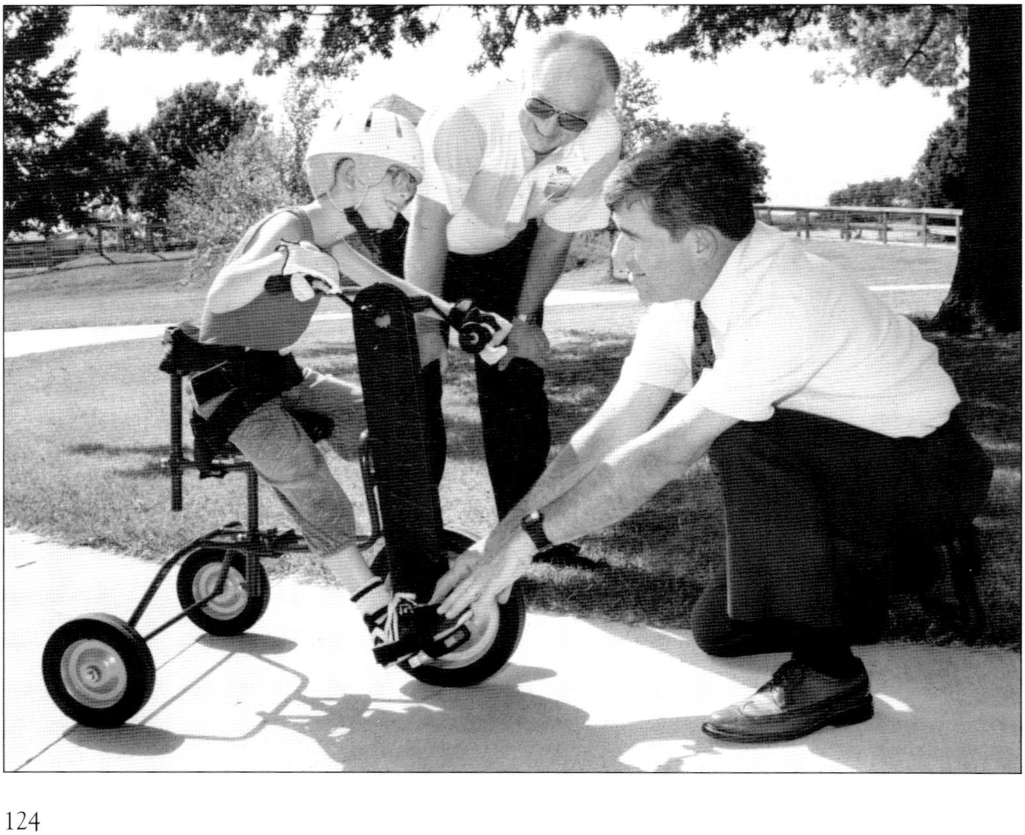

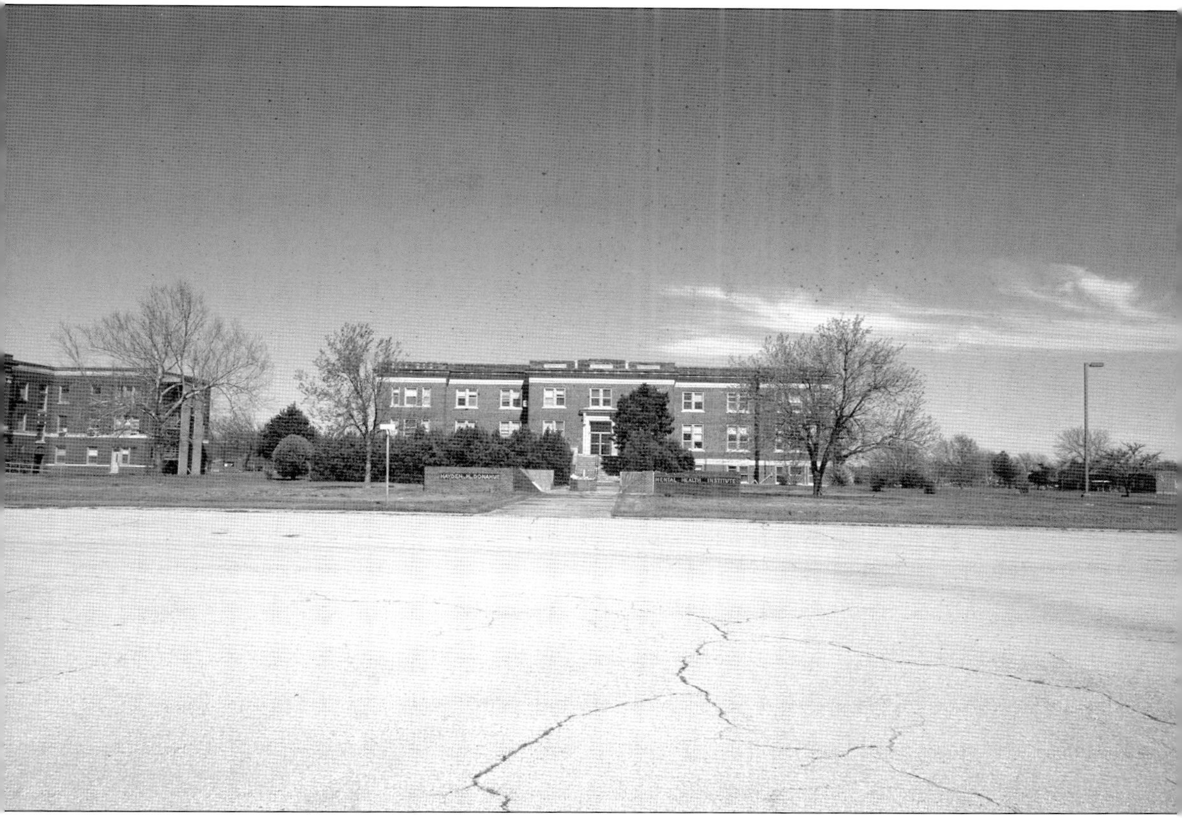

The original High Gate College, subsequently the Oklahoma Sanitarium Company administration building, burned down in 1926. The building pictured here, the current administration building, was erected after the fire. Today's lonely campus is the result of deinstitutionalizing and treating patients on an outpatient basis through community health care centers. But for many patients, the transition was not an easy one. Little forethought was given to the outcome of releasing long-term patients into mainstream society. Frank Keating, who became governor of Oklahoma in 1995, believed that most patients could be released into society and instructed Eastern State Hospital to start releasing those who could leave the hospital and work on their mental health with counseling at community health care centers. Many of those released from Eastern State Hospital could not adjust to life outside of the institution; they had high suicide rates, and emergency rooms were swamped with former patients who had no place to go. A lot of them had no other choice but to live on the streets. (CCHS.)

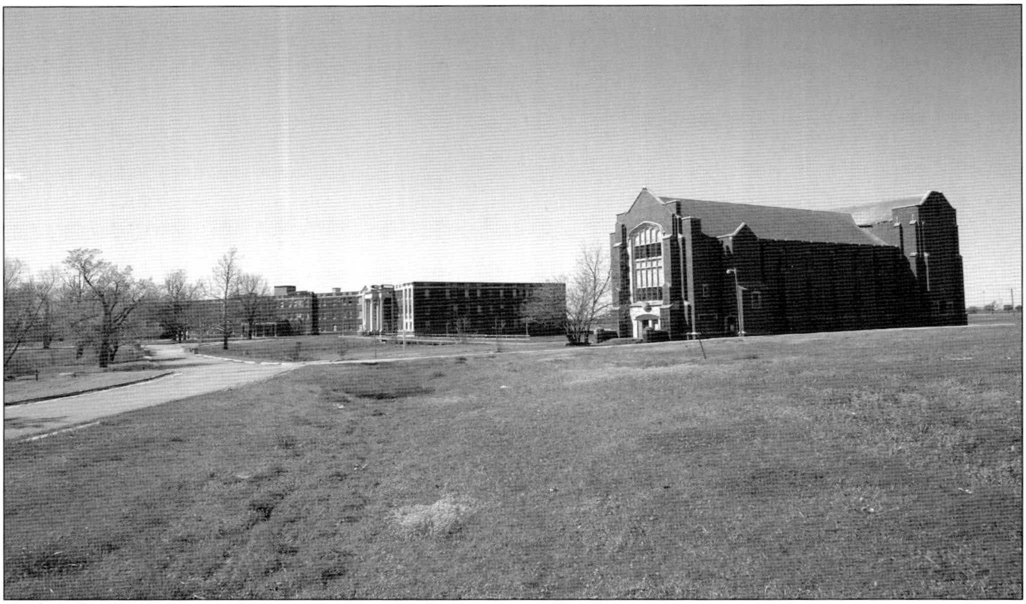

Two significant buildings on Griffin Memorial Hospital grounds still grace the campus today: Hope Hall and the American Legion Memorial Chapel. Hope Hall's main building was constructed in 1929, and two wings were added in 1930; altogether, the building had 100,000 square feet of space for the admission, evaluation, and housing of patients. (CCHS.)

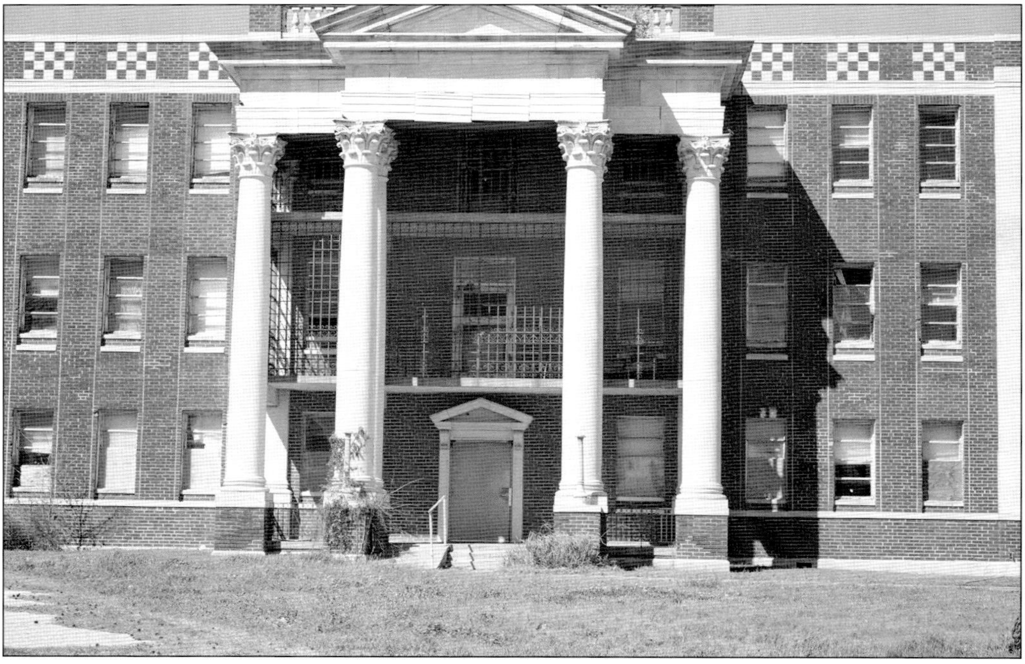

Today, the tall white columns that adorn the east and west wings of Hope Hall are crumbling, and the ornate bars that enclosed the secure ward on the upper floors are rusting. The "secure" wards were not only for violent patients but were also used by Norman and Cleveland County officials to house criminals until their court appearances. (CCHS.)

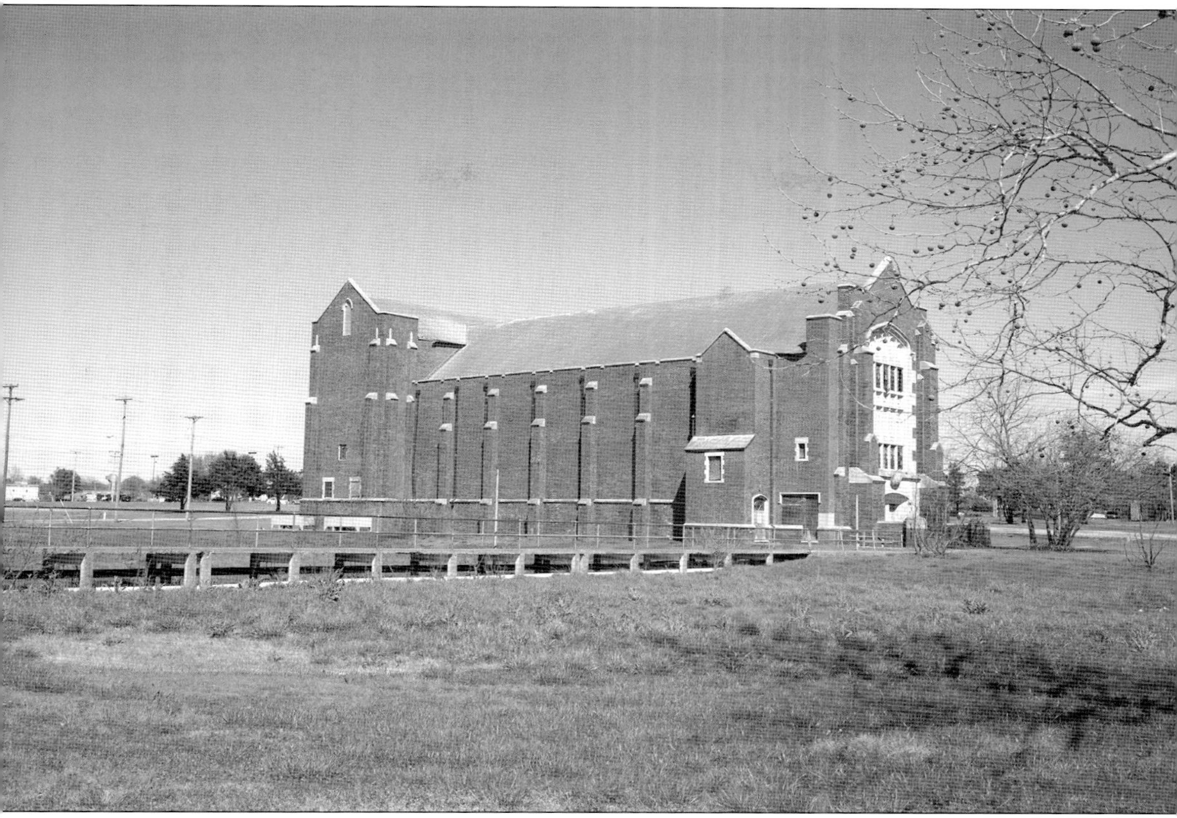

The American Legion Memorial Chapel is perhaps the most admired of the Griffin Memorial Hospital buildings. The chapel became exactly what Dr. David Griffin had intended it to be: a place where people could gather for entertainment and worship. Until the 1970s, a chaplain lived on the hospital grounds and conducted nondenominational services every week. Also, each Monday and Wednesday, the hospital band performed, and patients gathered at the chapel for square dancing. (CCHS.)